THE NATURAL WAY SERIES

Increasing numbers of people worldwide are falling victim to illnesses which modern medicine, for all its technical advances, seems often powerless to prevent – and sometimes actually causes. To help with these so-called 'diseases of civilization' more and more people are turning to 'natural' medicine for an answer. The *Natural Way* series aims to offer clear, practical and reliable guidance to the safest, gentlest and most effective treatments available – and so to give sufferers and their families the information they need to make their own choices about the most suitable treatments.

Titles in the Natural Way *series*

Allergies
Arthritis & Rheumatism
Asthma
Back Pain
Cancer
Candida
Chronic Fatigue Syndrome
Colds & Flu
Cystitis
Diabetes
Eczema
Epilepsy
Hay Fever
Heart Disease
HIV and AIDS
Infertility
Irritable Bowel Syndrome
Migraine
Multiple Sclerosis
Premenstrual Syndrome
Psoriasis

THE NATURAL WAY

Eczema

Sheena Meredith

Series medical consultants
Dr Peter Albright MD (USA)
& Dr David Peters MD (UK)

Approved by the
AMERICAN HOLISTIC MEDICAL ASSOCIATION
& BRITISH HOLISTIC MEDICAL ASSOCIATION

ELEMENT

Shaftesbury, Dorset ● Boston, Massachusetts
Melbourne, Victoria

© Element Books Limited 1994
Text © Sheena Meredith 1994

First published in the UK in 1994 by
Element Books Limited
Shaftesbury, Dorset SP7 8BP

Published in the USA in 1994 by
Element Books, Inc.
160 North Washington Street,
Boston, MA 02114

Published in Australia in 1994 by
Element Books
and distributed by
Penguin Australia Limited
487 Maroondah Highway, Ringwood, Victoria 3134

Reprinted 1995
Reissued 1998
Reprinted 1999

Cover Design by Slatter-Anderson
Designed and typeset by Linda Reed and Joss Nizan
Printed and bound in Great Britain

British Library Cataloguing in Publication
data available

Library of Congress Cataloging in Publication
Meredith, Sheena
The natural way with eczema/Sheena Meredith.
p. cm.
Includes bibliographical references and index.
ISBN 1-85230-493-6
1. Ezcema–Alternative treatment. 2. Naturopathy. I. Title
RL251.M47 1994
616.5′2106–dc20 94–25492
CIP

ISBN 1 85230 493 6

Contents

List of Illustrations

Introduction

Eczema and dermatitis are terms used to describe the symptoms of a certain kind of skin reaction that can have many possible causes. Sufferers range from tiny babies with an inherited tendency to angry outburts of raw, itchy skin which may never be traceable to any external factor, to elderly workers whose skin is dry, cracked and tired after years of 'abuse' from handling irritant substances. The two outstanding features which the various forms have in common are that they can create profound misery for those afflicted and for their families, and that they are often intensely resistant to treatment.

Modern medicine can be very effective in relieving symptoms of eczema but it cannot offer a cure. For many sufferers this means a life overshadowed by episodes of ugly, irritating and even painful skin. It may mean years of being dependent on skin creams or drugs to keep the skin manageable, or severe restrictions on the occupations, hobbies and social activities that can be pursued.

Not surprisingly, many patients are tempted by other forms of natural therapy – but it can be hard to know where to turn, which practitioners are reliable, or which treatments get results. This book aims to offer a guide to the many sources of help available: how they work, how effective they are, who provides them and what happens during consultations and treatment.

People generally turn to natural medicine after years of conventional treatment, and many find relief where conventional methods have failed. There are safe and effective treatments for eczema which offer a prospect of real improvement for more than four-fifths of patients, and almost everyone can expect to find something to lessen the frequency and severity of attacks.

Ultimately, however, the final responsibility for managing eczema lies - as it should - with the person affected, which is why this book also offers suggestions for practical self-help. You may always have sensitive skin. Cherish it, protect it, and seek help when you need it. Choose a therapy which suits your lifestyle, preferences and beliefs, because whatever it is it has a better chance of working if you start with a positive attitude. The suitability of a therapy is as important as its overall success rate, and it is up to you to get the best from whatever treatment you choose.

Sheena Meredith
Horton
England.

CHAPTER 1

What is eczema?

How skin works and why it goes wrong

Eczema is one of the most irritating, distressing and often unsightly skin conditions, having far-reaching effects on a sufferer's health, happiness and lifestyle. As many as one in ten people may be affected at some time in their lives, often in childhood, but the disease can also strike in adult life.

There are many types of eczema, all with similar symptoms. Areas of skin become dry, red and inflamed, often with scaly, flaky patches and sometimes with small blisters. These can weep, leading to crusting and scabs, or burst, leaving patches of raw skin. The skin itches constantly and may be sore.

Septic spots may develop if blisters become infected. Scratching can also encourage secondary infection, or cause dry, hard, thickened patches. In severe cases, especially if the sufferer has been scratching, raw or broken skin may bleed. Swelling due to fluid accumulation (oedema) may occur with eczema on skin which is loose or floppy, such as the eyelids or testicles.

All about skin

Skin is the main interface between us and our environment, so it is hardly surprising that it may be intimately affected by both our internal state (physical and psychological) and outside forces (infections, trauma or chemical attack).

Yet healthy skin is amazing stuff. It keeps out bugs, mud and bathwater, tolerates snow or tropical heat, stretches when we put on weight or become pregnant, then shrinks back to a perfect fit. It is self-repairing, rapidly healing cuts, scrapes and even surgical incisions, and every month its entire surface is renewed. Skin is regularly washed, rubbed, pinched and pummelled, and still stays soft and pliable enough to be nice to stroke. And even after up to a century of this punishing treatment the worst effects for most of us are the odd wrinkle and an age spot or three. No synthetic material could match this.

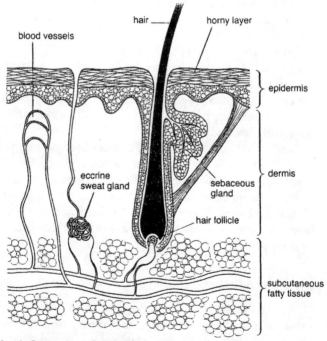

Fig. 1 Structure of the skin

Structure of the skin

Like all body tissues, skin is made up of tiny building blocks called cells. The outermost cells of the upper layer (or *epidermis*) form a tough, horny coating which protects against damage, disease, chemicals and other potential dangers, and largely (although not completely) prevents fluids leaking out or in. Despite its strength it is also elastic, enabling the skin to move and stretch. The cells of the horny layer are continually being shed from the skin surface (to create the vast majority of what we know as household dust), and gradually replaced by new cells pushing up from underneath them. As these lower cells move towards the surface, they produce a strong protein called keratin, which maintains the horny coat and forms the structure of hair and nails. In the course of their journey the cells die off - they are, in fact, dead when they are shed. Beauty may be skin-deep, but on the outside we are all dead dust-factories.

Normally it takes about 28 days for a cell to form, move to the surface and be shed, but the process speeds up if for any reason the surface layer is rubbed off - which is why some beauty experts recommend vigorous skin-brushing to remove dead cells and leave the skin looking shiny and new. Too much friction creates permanent thickening and toughening, as with a callous.

The skin pigment *melanin* is produced in the epidermis from specialized pigment cells with tentacle-like projections on their surface which inject melanin into the surrounding cells. Melanin filters out most of the harmful rays of the sun. Given time to swing into operation, the more they are exposed to the sun the more melanin the pigment cells produce. Too rapid an exposure, which does not give melanin time to accumulate, leads to sunburn.

Under the epidermis lies a stronger, thicker, layer of

skin called the 'dermis'. This is a tough, fibrous framework enclosing a supporting web of elastic fibres interwoven around hair roots and follicles, blood and lymph vessels, nerves and sweat glands. Ridges in the structure of the dermis are what create fingerprints.

The sweat-glands in the dermis are mostly a type called 'eccrine glands', which are widespread around the body. Together, they produce about half a litre of sweat each day, increasing their output by as much as ten-fold during exercise and in hot weather. Eccrine glands are also activated when we are under stress, which is why we get sticky palms just before an important meeting. Sweat evaporating from the skin surface cools it, a vital part of the body's temperature balance. The blood vessels of the dermis also open up in hot conditions, increasing their flow and bringing warm blood from the body's core to the surface, allowing it to cool down.

Another type of sweat-gland, the 'apocrine gland', is found in the hair follicles of the breasts, armpit and groin. These swing into action around puberty, producing a highly individual odour thought to be a crucial factor in sexual attraction, but with the potential to be unpleasantly smelly if allowed to go stale on the skin.

Opening into the hair follicles of the dermis are 'sebaceous glands' which produce sebum, the greasy material which lubricates the skin and protects against the elements.

The dermis has a rich supply of nerves which convey impulses from specialized endings called receptors to the brain, where the messages are interpreted as sensations of touch, pressure, heat, cold, itch or pain.

Damage to the skin

Despite its awesome adaptability and in-built protective mechanisms, the skin can be damaged by extremes of temperature (burns, frostbite), by trauma, chemicals, insect bites and radiation including sunlight. It may be affected by local skin disease or infection, or involved in bodily diseases and infections, such as chicken-pox. Adverse reactions to drugs and allergic responses often manifest in the skin.

In one recent survey, one-quarter of adults and more than a third of children had suffered from some form of skin complaint in the preceding two weeks.

Skin is more vulnerable in old age, when it is naturally drier, and during hormonal changes such as after childbirth and at the menopause. All skin diseases are more likely to take hold in someone who is poorly-nourished or anaemic, and symptoms are often made worse by stress and by extremes of temperature.

Skin reactions in eczema

The symptoms of eczema may stem from irritation of the skin, or allergy, or both. In either case, the basic reaction is one of inflammation, a process which arises in response to any attack on body tissues, whether from infection, injury or irritation (chemical or allergic). The skin cells release chemicals like prostaglandins which provoke inflammation and swelling (oedema). Specialized white blood cells called *lymphocytes*, part of the body's defence mechanisms, flood into the dermis from swollen and leaky blood vessels to try to deal with the attack. The area becomes swollen, red, hot and sore.

Irritation may follow trauma, drying out or chemical attack, and everyone is at risk although some people have more sensitive skin than others. An irritant reaction damages the horny layer and reduces its ability to defend itself against further damage. It also makes the skin vulnerable to penetration by substances likely to provoke allergic responses in susceptible people.

Allergic reactions

Allergies are an unfortunate by-product of the body's natural immune defences. Normally, when 'foreign' material such as germs or microbes (called 'antigens') enter the body, the immune system produces antibodies to neutralize them, so fighting off infection. An allergic person may produce antibodies to normally harmless substances, and the reaction between the antigen (now called an allergen) and its antibody stimulates special, highly reactive cells, called 'mast cells', to release chemicals such as histamine, which provokes an inflammatory response.

The exact symptoms of the allergy depend on where this occurs, so in the air passages it causes the wheezing of asthma, whereas in the skin it creates the intense itching of allergic eczema. It is estimated that as many as one in five people are allergic to something, and skin reactions are common.

Eczema or dermatitis?

There has been a long confusion between the terms eczema (from the ancient Greek meaning 'to boil over') and dermatitis (meaning 'inflammation of the skin'). Both refer to the same symptoms and in the USA all such reactions are more usually called dermatitis. In Britain, doctors traditionally labelled skin reactions to external substances as 'contact dermatitis' and reactions apparently generated internally (such as those due to food allergy) as 'eczema'. This distinction is fairly meaningless, however, and the terms eczema and dermatitis are often now used interchangeably. So if different doctors refer to your problem as 'atopic eczema' or 'atopic dermatitis' it's still the same condition.

Personal and social costs of eczema

People who have never had eczema or other skin diseases often think of them as trivial and superficial complaints, but sufferers and their families know all too well that they can have disastrous and debilitating effects.

Itching is one of the most annoying sensations, and when persistent can be more distressing than being in pain. Sufferers may become irritable and find they cannot concentrate, and the situation is often made worse by sleeping difficulty and chronic fatigue. Strained relationships and problems at school or work can result when the sufferer feels below par or bad-tempered and his or her performance is impaired.

Those with a prominent rash, especially on the face or hands, may be acutely aware of their skin and feel ugly and self-conscious as a result. This can be reinforced by other people's reactions. Although it is usually not deliberate, people do tend to hesitate or look embarrassed when they see someone who has an obvious skin problem. Strangers may back off or seem reluctant to shake hands, and some think (wrongly) that eczema is contagious and try to keep their children away from an affected child.

Sufferers can easily begin to feel that others are either staring at them or avoiding them. In severe cases, they may avoid going out, missing parties or social functions where they would have to meet new people, and shying away from sexual contacts. A vicious circle of loss of confidence and self-esteem, with difficulty making friends and forming relationships, can develop. Children with eczema may be teased or bullied in school, their school work may suffer and they may even develop a school phobia.

Adults often find that eczema interferes with their work or even limits their choice of occupation. A record of time off and having allergies to certain substances may affect future prospects. On a more subtle level, skin disease may mar someone's appearance and research has shown that, unfair though it is, attractive people tend to do better in many ways, from making a good first impression and attracting friends to getting on in their career.

The other side of the coin is that eczema, like many skin diseases, can be made worse by stress. Attacks may be precipitated or exacerbated by emotional problems, pressure at work or relationship difficulties.

Costs to the country

Eczema takes up a large proportion of doctors' time and resources. Skin conditions are the second most common reason (after respiratory - breathing - infections) for seeing a family doctor, accounting for about one in ten consultations. Eczema and dermatitis account for about half of all skin problems and up to one in five referrals to skin specialists.

Occupational dermatitis is one of the most common causes of lost working days to British industry and accounts for more than half of all compensation claims paid for industrial injuries.

Can eczema be cured?

A severe eczema sufferer is likely always to have sensitive skin and there is, at present, no 'cure' which can completely abolish this tendency. There are, however, many things people can do to reduce the risk of skin reactions, and many natural and gentle remedies (described in later chapters) which can help to clear up the skin and boost its defences against future attacks. With careful skin care, and by seeking appropriate treatment when necessary, most people with eczematous skin can reduce symptoms to manageable levels - for example with only occasional mild flare-ups when under stress. Many will achieve complete freedom from attacks, even though they may need to maintain constant vigilance about the substances they handle and a lifelong routine of good skin care - which has its own benefits.

CHAPTER 2

The different types of eczema

What they are and how they affect you

There are nearly a dozen different types of eczema but not all are as common or as widespread as each other. The most common are the contact eczemas and atopic eczema.

Irritant contact eczema

Skin may be traumatized by rubbing with abrasives like sandpaper or scouring pads, by repeated washing and drying which remove its natural grease, by cold or wind or extremely dry conditions which crack its surface, or by chemical irritants varying from industrial oils to household detergents.

Anyone is at risk of irritant contact eczema if this kind of rough treatment is sufficiently prolonged, although people vary considerably in susceptibility. Dry skin increases the risk, so reactions become more common with age as the skin dries out, and tend to be worse in winter. Fair-skinned redheads (the colouring most prone to sunburn) and people with other sorts of eczema, especially atopic eczema, are especially vulnerable.

Workers like mechanics who are always covered in oil, or hairdressers whose hands are continually wet or touching dyes and other hair products, often need time off to let the skin recover. In severe cases, the only relief may be by changing occupation.

Irritant Contact Eczema characteristics

- Most common form in adults, but can occur in children
- Causes most occupational or industrial skin problems
- Hands most often affected because most exposed
- May occur where clothing rubs (for example, armpit folds)
- Especially with strong detergents, oils, prolonged immersion
- Usually develops over a period of time
- May occur after one exposure to strong or caustic substances
- Years of minor wear and tear may lead to 'tired skin syndrome' with dryness and irritation
- May occur in babies
  - on the chin, due to dribble or encrusted food
  - one form of nappy rash

If irritant eczema does not clear up fairly rapidly it can spread to skin elsewhere, even parts which have not been in contact with the irritant substance. Once this has happened, the skin may remain hypersensitive for many years, and even minor damage can produce a widespread reaction. Very rarely, this leads to an extremely distressing and potentially dangerous condition called generalized exfoliative dermatitis or erythroderma, which affects the whole body.

Allergic contact eczema

This is less common but very similar to irritant eczema, although it may be more severe and develop much more rapidly after contact with the offending allergen. Almost every substance known has been incriminated but some provoke reactions more easily than others. Base metals are often involved, especially nickel, to which up to 10 per cent of young women are sensitive. Other common culprits include sticking-plasters, cosmetics, plants, rubber, glues, dyes and resins.

Allergic Contact Eczema characteristics

- Usually affects adults
- May be provoked or made worse by stress or strong emotions
- Diagnosis by patch-testing (see p. 26, 45)
- Sufferers often react to more than one allergen

This type of allergy develops after a susceptible person becomes sensitized to an allergen. The first time the allergen penetrates the outer layer of the skin (through hair follicles, sweat-ducts or tiny cracks), it combines with body protein to form an antigen. In time, the immune system recognizes this antigen, and subsequent contact with the same allergen provokes a rapid inflammatory reaction. Sensitization can take months or even years to develop, hence the strange 'ability' of people to develop allergies 'out-of-the-blue' to substances they have handled for some time. Some people react to chemically similar substances without this initial contact (cross-sensitization).

Atopic eczema

This is part of a genetic trait (called 'atopy') in which people are vulnerable to eczema, asthma and hay fever ('allergic rhinitis'). Most affected children have a relative with one or more of these complaints. Sufferers have an inherited tendency to allergic responses involving a particular sort of antibody called immunoglobulin E (IgE), which attaches to mast-cells. Both they and many of their blood relatives (whether affected or not) have high levels of IgE in their blood stream.

Children with atopic eczema are hypersensitive to allergens which need not directly touch the skin (the word atopic comes from the ancient Greek for 'displaced'). It could be something the child has eaten, for example. It is not always possible to identify the culprits but the most common are house dust mite, pollens and cat or dog fur.

Atopic (inherited) Eczema characteristics

- Most common form in children (also called 'infantile eczema')
- More common in bottle-fed than breast-fed babies
- May start at 2-3 months or earlier, almost always by age 2
- Occasionally disappears but comes back later
- Tends to improve with age, usually gone by puberty
- Occasionally begins after puberty, may then be persistent
- Worse in cold weather, or sweaty, humid conditions
- Sudden temperature change can cause intense itch (for example, getting into a hot bath)
- Anger or stress may exacerbate
- Often improves around age five, but asthma or hay fever may then develop
- Asthma follows in up to half of sufferers, usually by school-age
- Hay fever may appear later
- Increased risk of other allergies: for example, urticaria (nettlerash)
- Atopic children often allergic to cows' milk

In babies itching and dry, rough skin may develop before the rash but, of course, they cannot say so, so the first signs may be rubbing the head and face, persistent crying, disturbed sleep or scratch-marks. The rash usually starts on the scalp, cheeks or nappy area and may spread to the neck, hands, arms, front of the legs and, occasionally, to the chest and back.

As the child gets older the eczema is more likely to spread. In toddlers and older children it is typically found on the wrists, inside the elbows, backs of knees and thighs, and may spread to the trunk.

The chance of a child being affected is roughly doubled if one parent is atopic, and increased about fourfold if both parents are atopic. Moreover, for reasons not yet clear, atopy seems to be becoming more common: 20 years ago about one in ten of the British population were thought to be atopic, half of them developing eczema. Today, nearly one-third of children have some atopic symptom before their eleventh birthday, and more than one in five have atopic eczema.

Seborrhoeic eczema

This name is used for two types of eczema, found in both children or adults, which are really quite different. Having had the 'childhood' version does not increase the risk of developing the adult one.

Childhood seborrhoeic eczema

This is often present in newborn babies as `cradle-cap', a mass of thick, brown-yellow, greasy scales on top of the scalp and sometimes on the forehead. Later in infancy, crusted patches, often with a red surround, may appear on the scalp, behind the ears, on the eyebrows, in skin-folds such as the under-arm or nappy area (a form of nappy rash) and occasionally on the trunk.

Childhood Seborrhoeic Eczema characteristics
- Not inherited
- Rarely bothers the baby, but parents often worried by the appearance
- May become infected if scratched
- Usually clears up on its own, almost always before age 2
- Becoming less common, for reasons unknown

Adult seborrhoeic eczema

This form features scaly, red, itchy spots on the face, especially the nose and eyebrows, the chest, back, neck, under-arm or scalp. It tends to be persistent.

Adult Seborrhoeic Eczema characteristics

- On scalp may look like dandruff
- Cause unknown but linked with overactive sebaceous glands and increased risk of skin infections, especially yeast

---

Nappy rash

Nappy rash, with red, sore, broken, inflamed and painful skin, sometimes with spots or blisters, is most often an irritant reaction to urine or stools, but may also be a form of atopic or seborrhoeic eczema. At root, however, it is caused by the nappy, and becomes more likely the longer a baby's sensitive skin is left to steep in the warm damp atmosphere of a nappy: 'No nappy, no nappy rash'.The groin areas affected gives clues to the type of nappy rash:

- At the back near the anus: may be a reaction to stools, especially in a baby with diarrhoea or threadworm infection
- At the front around the genitals, but not the skin folds and creases: may be irritation from urine, especially if not changed regularly or if the baby has sensitive skin
- At front and back but not in folds and creases, with 'terry' towelling nappies: may be a reaction to washing powder
- Buttock creases: brown-red spots suggest seborrhoeic eczema, which may also be present on scalp or elsewhere.

Nappy rash characteristics

- May be difficult to clear up
- Secondary fungal infections with 'candida' (thrush) are common: baby may have white patches of thrush in the mouth and the rash may spread into skin-folds and creases
- May be signs of eczema elsewhere on the body

Other (rarer) forms of eczema

Discoid eczema

This is also known as 'nummular eczema', and is characterized by red, itchy, weepy, coin-shaped patches. It sometimes occurs in young adults (especially females) who have had atopic eczema in childhood, sometimes in middle-aged men (when it seems to be linked with stress), and sometimes in elderly people, especially men, with dry skin. The patches readily become infected.

Eczema craquelé

This is also called 'asteatotic eczema' and is the dry skin seen in elderly people, especially those who are too ill or institutionalized to care for themselves properly. It occurs typically on the shins and lower legs in cold, windy weather. It stems from reduced *sebum* production and thinning skin caused by age.

Neurodermatitis

This shows in patches of skin subject to prolonged nervous scratching or rubbing. The skin becomes leathery, thick and itchy, increasing the desire to scratch. It occurs typically on the neck or arm in tense people. It may also occur after scratching areas of the body where there are other forms of eczema: it is known then as 'lichen simplex'.

Varicose eczema

This is also called 'stasis' or 'gravitational eczema'. Itchy, irritating patches form on the ankle near varicose veins (when it may be a warning sign of a varicose ulcer) or a previous thrombosis (clot) in the leg veins. Contact reactions may develop on top, and it may spread to the arms or elsewhere.

Light-sensitive eczema

This type of eczema, also known as 'photosensitive eczema', develops in response to sunlight and so occurs on exposed areas such as the face, neck, hands and arms. It may develop on top of some other form of eczema, in response to contacts, or as an internal reaction. It is common in young women who sunbathe or use sunlamps, often starting after sunburn. In older people it may be as a result of drugs and medicines which sensitize the skin to light. Chemicals in soaps and cleansers may also be light-sensitizers, as can some plants including parsnips, stinking mayweed and giant hogweed – so gardeners and ramblers beware.

Pompholyx

This is also known as 'vesicular dermatitis' or 'dyshidrotic eczema'. Its itchy blisters on the palms and soles often complicate some other type of eczema. It is at its worst in hot humid conditions and is sometimes associated with stress, contact sensitivity (especially to nickel) or fungal infection.

CHAPTER 3

Common causes and triggers of eczema

What they are and how to avoid them

The most obvious way to relieve eczema is to identify the irritants or allergens causing, or at least triggering, the symptoms and avoid them, but this may require considerable detective work. People often react to many substances, and more than one form of eczema can exist at the same time. For instance, an atopic child can still suffer with irritant or seborrhoeic eczema (and other skin conditions), and often an allergic reaction develops on top of a contact eczema caused by something else.

When a rash develops it is natural to try to think of any recent contacts with unusual substances, and this is often vital to pinpointing the cause. However, it can lead to a wrong conclusion. The contact could be coincidental, or the true cause could be another skin disease which mimics eczema. Examples are *psoriasis* (another scaly skin disease), reactions to drugs and medicines taken internally, insect bites (bed-bugs, *scabies*) which have been scratched, and occasionally scratching of the original rash of childhood infections like measles or *roseola* if other symptoms (such as fever) are minimal.

The range of substances capable of causing an irritant reaction is vast (even including water if the skin is soaked for long enough), and it is possible to be allergic to almost anything. Allergic responses can be sparked by minute amounts of allergen, and while they are most often due to recent contacts they can arise from substances which have been used for ages without trouble. It may be impossible to identify specific triggers of atopic eczema.

Common sources of contact allergies

- Base metals especially nickel (jewellery, watch straps, bra straps, metal buttons, buckles and fasteners, metallic threads, name tapes)
- Drugs and medicines including skin creams, sticking plasters
- Cosmetic products (make up, perfumes, soaps, deodorants, talcs, bubble bath)
- Household products (bleaches, detergents, wax polishes, washing powder)
- Epoxy resins, chemical stabilisers in plastics and rubber
- Dyes, inks
- Sunlight (photosensitive reactions)
- Sunscreen products
- Wool
- House dust mite
- Grass pollen
- Animal hair and feathers
- Plants (poison ivy, primula, ragweed, poison oak, chrysanthemums, celery)

Finding the culprit

The first question to ask is where is the rash? The site can give a good guide to contact reactions but is occasionally misleading. The scalp is resistant, so reactions may be seen on the forehead, around the eyes and ears instead. Reactions involving skin-folds, especially in the armpit where clothing may rub, are common. But if the whole of the armpit is involved the cause may be adult seborrhoeic dermatitis rather than contact.

People touch their faces, especially their lips, continually, often unconsciously, and products like hand cream or nail varnish (which rarely causes reactions on the nails as they are inert) may cause reactions there rather than on the hands. Sometimes the offending substance is transferred from another person: for example, facial rashes in men caused by women's make up, or reactions in the groin area due to spermicides or contraceptive diaphragms.

Site of eczema and possible causes

- Scalp, forehead: shampoos, hair-dyes, hats, headbands
- Ears: earrings, spectacle frames, hearing-aids, ear-drops, scalp applications
- Eyelids and around eyes: eye make-up, eye-drops, dusts and gases, scalp applications, soap
- Face, mouth: cosmetics, soap, toothpaste, foods, plants, nail-varnish, handcream
- Chin, neck: ties, necklaces, scarves, perfume, dusts
- Skin-folds (like armpit): clothes (fabric, dyes, washing powder), deodorants
- Hands, forearms: household cleaning materials, industrial oils, pets, plants, rubber gloves
- Wrists: bracelets, cuffs, dusts
- Trunk: clothing, rubber or elastic in underwear, metal buttons, jeans rivets or buckles
- Whole body: probably something swallowed, food or drug
- Genital area: loo paper, clothing, contraceptives, talcs
- Thighs: suspenders, materials carried in pockets
- Feet and ankles: socks, stockings, shoes (rubber, dyes, glues)

Are you using anything for it?

Even medicinal skin products can cause contact eczema. Indeed it has been claimed that they are responsible for up to one third of all cases. Lanolin (wool fat), a common cause of reactions, is often used as a base for creams and ointments. Other culprits include antiseptics, eye and ear-drops, antihistamine cream and local anaesthetic ointments. Remedies described as natural, herbal or additive-free can still produce allergies.

What is your job?

Certain jobs involve more risk of contact eczema than others, either because of handling potential irritants and allergens, or from trauma from abrasives or constant soaking. Those at risk include mechanics, engineers, hairdressers, building workers, miners, factory workers, nurses, food-handlers, greengrocers, photographers, carpenters, cleaners, painters, farmers and laboratory workers.

If you think something you handle at work is the culprit, ask yourself these questions – any yes answers point to an occupational cause:

- Is there anyone else at work with a similar problem?
- Does your skin improve at weekends and holidays?
- Is the rash on exposed areas (like hands and forearms) only?
- Is the right hand (if right-handed) worse than the left?
- Has the problem only developed since starting work?
- Does it improve when you avoid the suspected substance, wear protective clothing or use barrier creams?

What are your hobbies?

Contact with potentially troublesome substances such as glues, dyes, photographic chemicals and plants can occur at home as well as at work, and the link may not be immediately obvious. For instance, plant reactions may trouble keen cooks and ramblers as well as gardeners.

Sensitivity to primula is very common and may cause both eczema and *urticaria*, with swelling of the face.

Do you keep animals?

Pets, especially dogs, cats, birds, and other furry animals like guinea pigs or rabbits, are potential sources of problems for anyone with an allergic tendency. Both fur (or feathers) and shed skin (dander) are potential allergens, and the more contact with them the more likely is a reaction, especially in young children. If you have an atopic child, don't keep pets, or if you must, keep outdoor animals, preferably in a cage, where the child's exposure can be well-controlled, or non-furry creatures like fish, tortoises or lizards. Don't allow visitors to bring furry animals into the house either, as the allergens can lie around for some time after the animal has gone.

What happens at home?

Contact reactions to household products are extremely common, especially to household cleaners and washing powders. Those advertised as 'biological' or 'low-temperature' contain enzymes which are more likely to cause skin problems. Cosmetics and toilet articles are also often incriminated.

Are you using any new products, or has the formula of an old favourite been changed recently? Beware especially anything containing detergents (including apparently 'gentle' products like bubble-baths), perfumes or antiseptics. Medicated, scented, moisturized or any other kind of soap with something added can only add to the risk of irritants being present. Hypoallergenic make-up and toilet products merely avoid the most common allergens, so some people are still allergic to them.

If you think you might be allergic to eye make-up,

stop wearing it altogether for a few days (yes, it may be difficult, especially if your eyes are already red and puffy, but try using a stronger blusher and lipstick instead, and perhaps a bold eyebrow pencil – but pick products you already know are safe).

Dust is another household danger. The house dust mite is probably the most important allergen of all. These tiny creatures, fortunately invisible to the naked eye, thrive in our modern warm houses, especially in mattresses and bedding: millions may live in a double-bed. They are also found in carpets, cushions, soft furnishings and children's cuddly toys. They feed mainly on shed scales of human skin, and their droppings (rather than the mites themselves) cause allergy in many of their human benefactors, especially those who already have eczema, because the mite products may then be scratched into already sensitive skin. Atopic children are particularly likely to be sensitive, often experiencing intense itching at night, and the tiny faecal particles ('droppings') can also provoke asthma or hay-fever if inhaled.

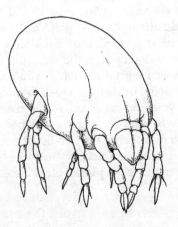

Fig. 2 The house dust mite

Playing detective

Quite often, eczema sufferers (and their doctors) run through all the most likely causes of a contact reaction and still draw a blank. Don't despair, there are still things you can do:

- Try avoiding common irritants and allergens as much as possible: change your washing powder, use hypo allergenic makeup, don't mend the car, use rubber gloves for washing up
- Carry a notebook everywhere you go and list everything you come into contact with, noting the dates of eczema flare-ups to try to spot any link
- Avoid any suspect substance for at least two weeks. If your skin gets better, reintroduce it cautiously to see if it makes the skin worse again. This is known as a 'challenge test'.

However, these trial-and-error procedures can be time-consuming and frustrating unless you strike lucky early on. If you have a contact allergy you could ask your doctor whether it is worth having a patch test (see chapter 5). Or you could attempt a d-i-y patch test yourself. Put a tiny amount of any suspicious substance on a small piece of gauze and stick it to the skin (the forearm is a good place to use) with a plaster (if you are allergic to plaster use sellotape or medical tape). Remove it after 48 hours, and if you find an eczema-type reaction underneath you may be allergic to that substance. Do not test substances you don't normally handle, or you could provoke a new sensitization, and if you feel a severe reaction is developing take the plaster off at once.

Atopic eczema

Since atopic eczema is an internally-generated response, and affected by emotions or temperature, pinning down specific allergens can be especially difficult. Monitoring what children get up to is difficult enough at home, and you need to know in detail what happens at school or friends' houses as well - a 'forgotten' helping of ice-cream at a birthday party, stroking a friend's pet mouse, or handling plants on the school botany outing could be critical.

If you suspect food allergy, you might need to keep a food diary for several months to spot any pattern between what the child eats and the frequency or severity of attacks. Checking your suspicions takes time too: it may take three weeks or more of eliminating (excluding) a particular food before any improvement occurs. Never make radical or long-term changes to a child's diet without first checking with your doctor, dietician or nutritionist as there is a risk of nutritional deficiencies.

Avoiding irritants and allergens

Some people are 'lucky' enough only to react to substances encountered in particular circumstances, like hair dyes or cement. But even then you need to beware of the same constituents turning up unexpectedly elsewhere. Others react to ingredients present in an often bewildering variety of products, and avoidance calls for constant vigilance. For example, it is amazing how many packaged foods contain milk or milk-products, such as skimmed milk powder or whey.

As well as avoiding as far as you can anything you have found to be a specific trigger for your eczema, it is a good idea to beware of other substances known to be commonly irritant or allergenic, because your skin is more likely to be vulnerable, especially if you are atopic.

Hints and tips on avoidance

- Always check labels for constituents
- Re-check labels, especially anything described as, for example, 'new, improved recipe': formulations can change
- Rinse skin and clothing thoroughly after washing
- Avoid strong detergents and 'biological' washing powders
- Keep a record of the household products you use, and note whether reactions relate to new ones
- Try changing brands of washing powders and cosmetics. Switch to the simplest, plainest soap you can find
- Test new cosmetics, shampoos, and so on on a patch of unobtrusive skin (like the arm) before using on the face or hair
- Wear only cotton next to the skin, especially if atopic – it's softer and lets the skin breathe
- If you suspect food allergy in an atopic child, use fresh foods and additive-free products as much as possible, and see whether avoiding dairy products helps
- In infantile eczema, avoid soaps, bubble-baths (even if special baby ones) and baby-wipes for a few days and wash with water only: mild cases may clear in a few days

---

Many people benefit from general measures to reduce common allergens like dust, mould-spores, plant and animal products, and this is particularly valuable for atopic children, where other triggers may remain a mystery. The house dust mite is the main allergen to control because it is strongly linked with eczema – as well as asthma and allergic rhinitis – and young children spend most of their time in the house. It may also help to prevent respiratory problems later.

Dealing with dust

- Damp-dust and vacuum the house at least once a week
- Concentrate especially on the bedroom, where children spend most of their time and which has the highest concentration of mites
- Arrange furniture, ornaments and toys to avoid dust-collecting areas which are difficult to clean
- Keep toys and clothes in chests, drawers and cupboards
- Remember textured wall-coverings, hanging mobiles, picture or clock-frames and plants also harbour dust
- If a child shares a room with brothers or sisters, treat all the beds in the room (or the mites simply move from one to another)
- Avoid bunk-beds, or give the child with eczema the top one
- Vacuum especially around and under the bed, and vacuum the mattress regularly
- Choose a bed with feet rather than one that rests on the floor, so you can clean underneath
- Ordinary vacuum-cleaners which beat the carpet can stir up more dust than they clean up, and they do not filter small particles like house dust mite from the exhaust air. Try to use an efficient cleaner with special exhaust filters, preferably one which can wet-wash the carpet
- Wash sheets and blankets or duvets regularly (ideally weekly) at a temperature of at least 55°C to kill mites
- Choose curtains which can be washed in the same manner, or have a roller blind instead – but not venetian blinds which are difficult to dust
- Use cellular blankets and polyester-filled duvets and pillows
- Hang sheets, blankets and duvets outside to air whenever possible (in many continental towns bedding is hung over the balcony every morning)
- Put pillows in the freezer overnight to kill off mites
- Try to stop the child taking furry toys to bed, or limit to special favourites, wash weekly and leave in the freezer overnight afterwards

- Use wooden or plastic chairs rather than upholstered ones
- Have bare floorboards or lino rather than carpets. Fitted carpets are the worst - choose a short pile one if you must, and synthetic fabrics rather than wool – or have rugs over a hard floor and clean them regularly
- Never shake rugs, blankets, duvets and so on indoors
- Maintain a good circulation of air with windows open whenever weather permits, and have at least a small window open at night – but keep windows closed during the day in the pollen season.

Special measures

- Chemical insect-killers may help, but killing the mites does little good if their droppings remain, so clean thoroughly at the same time. Remember that these chemicals can also be irritant to eczema sufferers
- Special mite-proof covers for bedding are efficient but expensive. Make sure they are permeable, otherwise they trap body heat and sweat and make eczema worse, and have wipe-down surfaces for easy cleaning
- Some manufacturers incorporate special barrier materials into new bedding to stop mites getting into the mattress
- Non-allergenic pillows and duvets only mean the filling should not provoke allergies - they are just as liable to become home to a large colony of mites unless covered with special barriers or washed regularly

Other hints

Other measures which may help against eczema are to avoid stirring up the air and creating damp atmospheres. Both these increase the concentration of dust and other allergen particles such as pollen or mould-spores in the air. Also

- Don't use fan heaters – but high efficiency air-filters and air-conditioners may help
- Avoid humidifiers

- Don't allow food to lie around going mouldy
- Treat any damp in the house promptly
- Fit extractor fans in kitchens and bathrooms to limit condensation
- Try not to live near rivers, canals or waterlogged ground.

Case history

Tom is four and has had severe eczema on his trunk, limbs and face since he was a baby, making him irritable and keeping him and his family awake at night. His mother is a doctor, so they had tried most medical treatments. But while she could soothe his symptoms she could not stop them from flaring-up time and time again. Eczema runs in the family, and one day her sister-in-law, who has it too, pointed out how dusty Tom's room was. She set to, wet-dusting from top to bottom, including all the areas people often forget – tops of picture-rails, paintings and window-frames. She vacuumed his mattress and under his bed, washed all his bedding and curtains at a high temperature, and took out his fluffy toys.

Tom's eczema began to improve, so his mother stuck to a rigid weekly cleaning routine. Within three weeks Tom's eczema had almost completely cleared up: "I was amazed. I knew about regular dusting and so on – I tell all my patients with eczema to do it. But I thought for it to make any difference I'd have to clean the whole house like that and I just don't have time. I couldn't believe the improvement from just keeping his bedroom clean and taking out all the furry animals."

CHAPTER 4

How to help yourself

You can do a great deal to help yourself if you suffer from eczema – even if you cannot 'cure' the problem. Obviously you should first be sure that you really have eczema (check with your doctor if in any doubt), and preferably find the triggers and so avoid them whenever possible (see chapter 3). You can also protect your skin to reduce the chance of repeat attacks. Children with atopic eczema need special care not only to help their eczema but also to reduce the risk of later respiratory problems. A careful routine of skin care is vital for everyone to aid healing and make the skin as robust and healthy as possible so it can defend and heal itself. Lastly, however hard you try, eczema is a long-standing condition. All kinds of unexpected things can cause a flare-up, and getting together a home survival kit to combat troublesome symptoms can be a huge reassurance.

Skin care and protection

Dry, cracked, chapped or broken skin is particularly at risk from eczema, and even between attacks your skin needs special care and attention.

Moisture cream helps prevent dryness, not by adding fluid but by stopping what is there escaping. Use it every time you have finished washing (preferably while the skin is still slightly damp) especially in cold, windy or sunny weather. Hand-creams are vital too, and you may find a plain emollient – a cream or ointment which soothes, moisturizes and helps prevent dryness – offers extra protection. There is no need for expensive products making extravagant claims. Simple, cheap ones will do the job just as well.

If your skin is very dry and using soap makes it worse, use a substitute such as an emollient aqueous cream. Try an emollient bath additive, or a water softener, which reduces the amount of soap needed for washing. There is little evidence, however, that expensive water-purification systems have an effect on eczema.

Gentle exposure to sunlight may help, but avoid extremes of temperature as sweaty conditions can make it worse. Avoid tight clothing and synthetic fabrics, especially for underwear.

Eczema is a good excuse for getting out of washing-up, as immersion for too long can cause dry, cracked skin. You should also avoid abrasive cleaners and scouring-pads. Limit soaks in the bath to no more than 15 minutes.

If you must do wet work, use abrasives or handle potentially irritant substances, always wear gloves and use a good barrier cream on your hands. This forms a partial shield against water and irritants, and makes the skin easier to clean. Cotton gloves, or PVC lined with cotton, are best. Rubber gloves make the skin soggy and vulnerable if worn for long periods, so wear absorbent cotton gloves underneath to minimize sweating.

Do not:

- Scratch
- Burst blisters (you risk introducing infection)
- Use unnecessary products such as bubble-bath (which dries the skin): bath oils are better

- Put disinfectant in the bath – ever
- Over-wash until the skin becomes dry
- Use over-the-counter eye-drops for allergies to eye-makeup
- Have your hair or eyelashes dyed: permanent products can cause long-lasting reactions.

Skin care products

Soap substitutes
- Wash E45: washing cream of zinc oxide and mineral oils
- Aqueous cream BP (emollient) or emulsifying ointment BP

Bath products
- Bath E45: unperfumed bath oil based on mineral oils
- Savlon bath oil: liquid paraffin and wool alcohols
- Hydromol emollient: bath additive containing liquid paraffin
- Oilatum emollient: bath additive with liquid paraffin
- Oilatum gel: shower gel with liquid paraffin

Emollients and barrier creams
- Aqueous cream BP
- Emulsifying ointment BP
- Cream E45: petroleum jelly, liquid paraffin, lanolin
- Eczederm cream: calomine and arachis oil (not for children)
- Oilatum cream: arachis oil (lanolin-free)

Occupational eczema

If your job involves handling substances which bring on your eczema your skin needs extra tender loving care, both for its own sake and for that of your job.

After an acute reaction, you need time away from the offending substances for the skin to heal. Bandaging may enable you to do dry work while the eczema clears up. For most people with irritant dermatitis, scrupulous skin-care and protection enables return to normal work, although relapses may occur. Use barrier cream under gloves before each handling, but do not be misled into assuming that this forms a total barrier over the skin. Other protective measures are needed as well:

- Beware rubber gloves – some solvents penetrate them, and some people are allergic to rubber
- Cotton-lined PVC gloves are best, but may make fine hand movements difficult
- Change and wash gloves (and other protective clothing) frequently, or use disposable plastic gloves
- Do not use solvents to remove oils: they may do more damage than the oils themselves
- Rings (and watches or bracelets if your wrists are exposed) can trap irritants and impede washing and drying - take them off at work
- Dusts stick to moist skin (such as the groin and armpit) so shower or bathe after working in a dusty atmosphere, or as soon as you get home

If these measures fail and you still suffer from eczema, talk to your family doctor or occupational physician, to your supervisor or union representative. Often changes can be made so that you can use different substances, avoid certain jobs or transfer to a different part of the factory or a different job within the same company. The aim is not to stop work but to find work which does not aggravate the eczema.

However, people with allergic contact dermatitis – about one in seven cases – *must* avoid the sensitizer (the substance that causes the eczema) because they will always develop eczema on the slightest contact, and this may necessitate a change of job.

Children with eczema

One of the most difficult tasks for a parent is to stop a baby or small child with eczema from scratching, which many do even in their sleep. It can cause dry leathery skin, especially around the neck and in the folds of elbows and knees. Keeping the eczema covered by bandages or clothing helps, as does keeping the child's nails short and clean, and wearing mittens in bed. But never – *ever* – be tempted to tie the child's hands to the cot. It is cruel and potentially dangerous.

Many mothers feel guilty or worry that eczema shows a lack of cleanliness (it doesn't). Consequently they tend to overdo washing which risks drying out the skin. It is even more important with a child's delicate skin to avoid soaps. Substitute an emulsifying ointment, and use an unperfumed emollient cream afterwards to help dryness and itching. Also use cream at bedtime and on exposed areas before going outdoors in cold or windy weather.

It also helps to keep room temperatures constant, not too hot or too cold, nor too dry or damp. Avoid sudden temperature changes, like getting into a hot bath in a cold bathroom.

Liaising with school
Do explain to the class teacher if a child has eczema, and check with both child and teacher that the child is not being bullied or ostracized because of the skin condition. The teacher can keep an eye out for the child and if necessary explain to other children and parents that eczema is not catching (contagious). You may also need the teacher's help with avoiding suspect allergens, especially foods, animals (like the class guinea-pig), and plants in the grounds or on school outings. The teacher can help by not sitting the child next to a radiator or a window, and reinforcing the importance of good skin-care.

Preventing complications of atopic eczema
If you are atopic, the most effective way to prevent your children being affected is to breast-feed them. Atopic eczema is some seven times more common in bottle-fed

than breast-fed babies. Breast-feeding is thought to be protective because breast milk both offers immune protection and contains substances such as *gamma-linoleic acid* (GLA) which may relieve eczema (see chapter 9). Children with atopic eczema are often allergic to cows' milk protein (and vice versa), and the later you can delay their exposure to it the less likely is the risk of a reaction.

Children suffering from atopic eczema are also at risk later of asthma and 'hay fever' – a combination of *allergic rhinitis* (a runny nose) and *allergic conjunctivitis* (red, itchy, streaming eyes), especially in spring and summer. It makes sense to try to protect their air passages and lungs as well as their skin. Do not smoke around them, as many of the substances in tobacco-smoke are extremely irritating to people with sensitive eyes, noses or lungs, and may increase the risk of asthma. If you must smoke in the house confine your tobacco to one room – preferably one with good ventilation – which the children do not enter. Similarly, you may not wish to be rude to guests who smoke but most smokers understand a request only to smoke in the smoking room, especially with a child in the house.

For the same reason avoid solid fuel (coal or wood) or paraffin for heating or cooking wherever possible. Electricity is much cleaner. Make sure that any appliances you do use are well vented and check the vents regularly.

Very rarely, children with atopic eczema develop an extreme and potentially dangerous reaction to *herpes* viruses – the cause of cold sores and genital herpes (other infections such as measles often improve more quickly in atopic eczema sufferers, for reasons unknown). This is known as 'eczema vaccinatum' and, in days gone by, also occurred with smallpox virus infection or vaccination, but fortunately smallpox has now disappeared and vaccination against it is obsolete.

It is worth ensuring that anyone with obvious cold sores does not kiss your child (even at the risk of causing offence to doting relatives).

To vaccinate or not to vaccinate?

Although in the past doctors tended to avoid giving certain immunizations, particularly tetanus, while a child had active eczema, most now believe this precaution is no longer necessary with modern methods of vaccine production. The conventional view is that children with eczema should generally receive all the standard immunizations because, as for other children, the benefits of protection against disease outweigh the risks involved. However, among natural therapists there is more of a debate about the potential long-term hazards of immunizations in general (see p. 115-16), and some parents remain anxious. If you are in any doubt discuss it with your doctor or some other medically-qualified practitioner.

Children with atopic eczema are sometimes accused of hyperactivity, and this is sometimes put down to an allergic reaction to a variety of environmental factors including sugar, additives, dairy produce, citrus fruits, environmental pollution, fluoride, aluminium and car exhaust fumes. However it may be some comfort to harrassed parents that atopic children tend to be of above average intelligence. They are typically inquisitive, alert, active, need little sleep and are highly responsive to their environment – a fact which may make them seem oversensitive at times. It is important not to label such children as abnormal just because they need a lot of stimulation, nor to be over-protective in restricting their diet or activities.

Nappy-rash

The ultimate cure for nappy-rash is to leave the nappy off. Try to give the baby some time with the skin exposed to fresh air – outside in the garden in the summer, inside on a towel in the winter or, with toddlers, in a room with a lino or tiled floor.

Change nappies frequently, and as soon as stools are detected. Wash the skin thoroughly with plain, warm water and use a good barrier-cream each time (such as zinc and castor oil or kamillosan cream). Use a thickish layer but not so much it makes a sticky patch on a disposable nappy or it may not absorb urine so well. If you use terry towelling nappies try to switch to disposable ones for a while. If you cannot afford this leave off plastic pants, switch to a mild washing powder and make sure you rinse it out well. If there is a secondary infection it may help to soak terry nappies in antiseptic during each wash, but again be sure to rinse thoroughly afterwards.

Products for nappy rash

- Zinc and castor oil cream: as barrier cream for regular use, and for treatment
- Savlon nappy rash cream
- Sudocrem antiseptic healing cream (contains lanolin)
- Vasogen cream: contains calamine for itching
- Vaseline pure petroleum jelly: for prevention only
- Kamillosan ointment: chamomile extract, helps soreness
- Morsep cream: vitamin A and cetrimide, emollient
- Canesten or Daktarin creams: for infected nappy rash (suspect if the rash does not clear despite other treatment)

Relief for eczema symptoms

There are a number of simple remedies available from your chemists which can help in an acute attack of eczema. Topical steroid creams contain *hydrocortisone* and should not be used for children under ten without medical advice. Those available without prescription are for irritant and allergic contact dermatitis only, and should not be used in pregnancy or on the face or genital area. If you wish to use them, apply sparingly *only* on the affected area. Do not put a bandage on top, and never use for more than seven days. If the skin does not improve rapidly, see your doctor. For a fuller discussion of *antihistamines* and *steroids* see chapter 5, pp. 47-9, 50-1.

In addition, various simple herbal remedies can be bought or prepared at home (see chapter 9, p. 109). If your eczema seems to be brought on or made worse by stress, you may find some of the relaxation techniques described in chapter 7 helpful.

Products to help eczema symptoms

- Two tablespoons sodium bicarbonate in a warm bath helps skin irritation
- Calamine helps itching but needs to be applied frequently. Available as cream, ointment or lotion, and in an emollient base with arachis oil (Eczederm)
- Evening primrose oil or borage (Starflower oil) capsules may relieve inflammation (see chapter 5). Do not use on children under seven without your doctor's advice
- Potter's skin eruptions mixture, a herbal remedy traditionally used to relieve symptoms in mild eczema (for adults and children over eight only)
- Morhulin ointment: contains zinc oxide and cod liver oil, useful for eczema and nappy rash
- Gelcosal: helps clear skin-scaling
- Infantile seborrhoeic eczema: rub with olive oil then wash with ordinary baby shampoo or special products like Dentinox cradle cap treatment shampoo
- Adult seborrhoeic eczema: Gelcotar or Polytar liquids, hair treatments or shampoos containing selenium to help 'dandruff'
- Light-sensitive reactions: Spectraban or Sun E45 lotion and cream absorb the (invisible) wavelengths of sunlight

which most often damage the skin, and are available in various strengths
- Antihistamine tablets help relieve itching, especially if disturbing sleep. May be useful for symptoms of both eczema and hay fever:
  - Aller-eze (adults and children over three only)
  - Seldane tablets (adults only)
  - Triludan (adults and children over six only)
  Avoid antihistamine creams for eczema as they can cause hypersensitivity and make the reaction worse (but may be useful in urticaria)
- Topical steroid creams available without prescription:
  - Dermacort cream
  - HC45 hydrocortisone cream
  - Lanacort creme
  - Lanacort ointment
  - Eurax HC: crotamiton and hydrocortisone

Ionization

Negative ions are charged particles found in the air naturally by the sea and waterfalls and after thunderstorms. They account for the refreshing and invigorating feelings of taking a walk by the sea, or even a shower. Conversely, the atmosphere before a storm may make us feel tense or miserable because the air is depleted of negative ions. Air pollution can have the same effect, as can modern houses or offices with central heating, air conditioners, synthetic fabric furnishings and carpets and a profusion of electrical appliances. This is believed to increase the risk of a variety of symptoms including allergies and asthma.

Ionizers, small machines which produce a flow of negative ions, seem to help people with respiratory problems such as bronchitis, sinusitis, asthma and hay fever – partly through an effect on body chemicals and partly by drawing dust-particles out of the air, including small fibres and cigarette-smoke which may irritate the air passages. Many people have also found they help conditions such as migraine, depression and eczema – although quite why and how they do is less clear. There are no known side-effects, although the ions can produce ozone in the air which may act as an irritant to some asthmatics.

Buying an ionizer is a relatively cheap experiment, and may be especially worth a try if you use a lot of electrical equipment such as videos and home computers, if you smoke or if you are sensitive to dust (use especially after releasing a sudden cloud when dusting, vacuuming or changing beds).

The ionizer should be positioned at least 20 inches away from walls and furniture to allow a free flow of air, and within six feet of the bed at head level at night. Although it makes the air cleaner it draws particles towards it and because deposits tend to settle on walls and furniture nearby as a result you need to clean more often.

Other sources of help in the UK

- National Eczema Society (see Appendix A)
- The Employment Medical Advisory Service (EMAS): offers free advice on occupational health problems to both employers and employees. Your local department is listed in the telephone book under 'Health and Safety Executive'
- Occupational dermatitis may entitle you to claim for disability benefit under the DHSS Industrial Benefit Scheme. For help or advice, talk to your supervisor or union representative, or to 'Disability Alliance' (see Appendix A)

- Your local chemist: pharmacists can advise on skin care, products available without prescription, and when to seek medical help for something stronger
- Prescription charges: if you need multiple items on repeat prescriptions you can reduce the cost by buying a 'season ticket'. Ask for leaflets in your local post office
- Under the 'Aids for Handicapped Persons' rules, people with asthma, dust allergies and eczema can buy certain goods such as special vacuum-cleaners VAT-free. Ask your supplier for details.

When to seek further advice

- If a new rash does not clear up in a few days
- If in any doubt about what it is
- If it covers a large area
- If it oozes or weeps a lot, especially in a child
- If it gets worse despite self-help measures
- If it comes back after successful treatment
- If treatment has no effect
- If nappy rash does not clear within a few days or if signs of thrush (white patches) are found in the mouth.

CHAPTER 5

Conventional treatments and procedures

What your doctor is likely to say

Unless the cause of your problem is fairly obvious your family doctor will probably ask a series of questions to find out about the rash, about you and your circumstances, and about your personal and family medical history. If you have any ideas yourself about what may be causing the skin reaction say so.

Most patients with skin disease try to clear it up themselves before seeing a doctor – yet many skin creams and lotions cause skin reactions so the doctor's job can be complicated if you are not truthful about what you have already used.

The doctor will examine your skin – not necessarily just the site of the rash, as sometimes other areas are affected without the patient noticing or realizing the connection. For instance, a rash on the hands is often accompanied by one on the feet.

Diagnosis

Sometimes eczema can be diagnosed fairly easily – for example, in a child from an atopic family with a typical skin rash or if someone has just started making model aeroplanes using epoxy glues. Often, however, the diagnosis is less clear-cut.

Since skin conditions develop and change with time, and often do not fit text-book descriptions, monitoring them for a while often helps. 'Come back if it's not better next week' is not an unreasonable approach – but do make another appointment if the rash has not disappeared.

You may be asked to adopt avoidance measures (see chapter 3) to see if this makes any difference, or to keep a diary of symptoms and contacts to look for hidden links. If an allergic reaction is suspected, you may be referred to a skin clinic at the local hospital for special tests such as patch testing of the skin, or special diets to uncover food sensitivities *(see below)*. Occasionally a blood sample will be taken to look for antibodies in the bloodstream (a RAST test), but this is rarely performed nowadays as it is generally unreliable. Some doctors with an interest in clinical ecology use specialized tests for food sensitivity (see p. 91).

Patch tests

Patch testing involves deliberately putting potential allergens (either those already suspected, or a batch of common sensitizers such as fur, nickel or pollen) onto an unaffected area of skin, usually on the arm or back. Each site is marked with felt tip and covered with gauze and medical sticky tape or plasters for 24-48 hours, then the skin is examined again a couple of days later. A positive test produces an eczematous reaction at the site of the incriminated substance.

A special form of patch test may be used for light sensitive reactions, in which two patches of each suspected allergen are put on, and one is exposed to ultraviolet light.

Patch tests are fairly simple and effective in many patients but there are drawbacks, such as:

- Strong reactions with unbearable itching (remove the test patch early)
- Sensitization to new allergens
- False negative results: the person is really allergic but the test does not show it, because it does not exactly mimic real life contact

Elimination (or exclusion) diets

Conventional medicine does not place as much emphasis on food intolerance as does natural medicine, but it increasingly recognizes that diet may play a role in atopic eczema. Doctors with leanings towards nutritional medicine or clinical ecology (see chapter 8) will probably look for food intolerance in childhood eczema as studies have shown that it is implicated in at least a quarter of all cases.

If a cause cannot be readily identified by avoiding common allergens (especially dairy products), trial and error, or keeping a food diary, the classic way to uncover it is to put the patient on an 'elimination' or 'exclusion diet' *(see also chapter 8)*.

In its most extreme form, this involves eating only an excruciatingly boring selection of bland foods (classically lamb, rice, peeled pears and boiled tap-water) until the symptoms settle down (up to three weeks). Other foods are then re-introduced one by one, leaving a few days between each to allow for any symptoms to appear.

This should only be carried out under strict medical supervision which, for children, may mean admission to hospital. It can lead to a temporary flare-up of the allergy and withdrawal symptoms such as headaches, may not identify an allergy even if it is present, and can lead to new sensitivities because the non-restricted foods are consumed in larger quantities than usual. Many doctors prefer to avoid it unless the patient is desperate, for obvious practical and humanitarian reasons. However less severe, modified versions have been devised for both children and adults.

Conventional treatment

Your doctor's advice on avoiding allergens and irritants, and on basic skin-care and protection, is likely to follow similar lines to that given in the previous two chapters, and sometimes these simple measures are all that is necessary.

In any more than the mildest case, you will probably be given specific treatment to help reduce symptoms and heal the skin, and other medicines as needed to treat secondary infections or aid sleep. If flare-ups seem to be triggered by stress, or if the problem is *neurodermatitis*, counselling or psychotherapy may be advised, or a short course of tranquillizers offered. In varicose eczema the doctor can arrange treatment of varicose veins (by injection or surgery) before ulcers develop.

Steroid creams

Corticosteroid drugs (often just called steroids) in the form of creams and ointments are the most common treatment for eczema. They are also known as 'topical steroids' (that is, they are applied directly to the skin unlike steroid pills which work internally).

These creams work by alleviating the symptoms of eczema, not by curing the condition. They reduce inflammation, so lessening redness, swelling and weeping, relieve itching and other symptoms, and allow healing of damaged skin. Initially you may be asked to apply the cream up to four times daily, and after prolonged use taper off gradually to once-daily or less as the condition improves. You should never stop treatment suddenly as this can lead to sudden relapse and worsening of the eczema.

While steroids are extremely effective in treating eczema, they should be used with caution (as your doctor will probably warn you). They may damage collagen protein in the dermis, and with over-use this can lead to skin thinning (which increases the risk of infection), striae (fine lines like stretch marks) and premature ageing. Other side-effects, especially with stronger preparations, may include:

- Acne or increased hair-growth
- Spread of untreated infection
- Some preparations contain potential skin sensitizers
- Bodily side-effects such as hormone imbalances if strong steroids are absorbed through the skin (very rare)
- Stunted growth in children.

Steroids should therefore be used sparingly and only on areas of skin affected by eczema, avoiding the vulnerable skin on the face and the genital region whenever possible.

Topical steroids are available in a variety of strengths, so the weakest capable of controlling the symptoms should be used for the shortest time necessary. Although you can buy weak preparations of hydrocortisone over the counter (for use by ten-year-olds or over), your doctor can prescribe from a much wider range suitable for different ages, sites or needs. For example, stronger preparations may be needed for the feet because the tougher skin absorbs less of the drug.

Sometimes you will be advised to use the cream under a dressing, or under a plastic bag or sheet of 'cling-film' overnight, which increases the amount of drug penetrating the skin and so enhances its effects (some people discover this useful tip about skin creams for themselves, but do not do it with steroids without your doctor's approval or you could overdose or damage the skin).

In general, if steroid creams are prescribed you will not need any additional topical treatments, and indeed other creams applied to already sensitive skin only increase the risk of further skin reactions. However, if a secondary infection has set in, or if the area of eczema is also affected by thrush (for example the nappy area or ear canal), combined preparations may be advised. Sometimes steroids are combined with tar preparations.

Very, very rarely – in severe cases – a doctor may advise steroid tablets, in which case they will be prescribed for as short a period as necessary to control the eczema, and withdrawn with great care for fear of precipitating a rebound reaction. Steroid tablets are used to treat the rare but dangerous complication *exfoliative dermatitis*. This is potentially fatal and so should always be treated in hospital.

Occasionally steroids may be injected into the skin if there is a local reaction which does not improve with topical steroids.

Tar-containing preparations

Coal-tar (as ointment, cream, paste or solution) soothes the skin, reduces itching and inflammation and may help to thin patches which are rough and thick from habitual scratching. It is especially useful for discoid eczema, in which topical steroids are less effective.

However tar paste is awkward to apply, messy, smelly, and stains clothing, so it is best used at night under bandages with old nightclothes and sheets. Preimpregnated bandages worn for a week or so are cleaner, and also stop scratching and can give a useful psychological boost by hiding the skin and giving an indication to colleagues that certain substances can't be handled.

Tar shampoos are useful for adult seborrhoeic eczema, and may be given with lithium ointment for the skin to reduce inflammation. Most tar preparations cannot be used on the face or on broken skin. Occasionally they can cause acne, contact or light-sensitive reactions.

Other topical preparations

- Zinc and calamine creams: help itching
- Potassium permanganate dressings or baths: help infected, weeping skin
- Ichthammol (shale) ointment or bandages: may help mild eczema
- Salicylic acid: may help thick, scaly skin (often used before tar preparations).

Antihistamines

Allergic responses involve the release of histamine and other itch-producing chemicals in the skin (see pp. 13-14), so using antihistamines to control itch is logical – although, of course, it does not prevent the allergic response from occurring in the first place.

Antihistamine creams are usually avoided (except for those with *urticaria*) because they can provoke skin sensitivity, but tablets may be prescribed to use either regularly in frequent allergic reactions, or before occasional exposures. Although people vary in their reactions, they tend to cause drowsiness, especially if taken with alcohol, so monitor your reactions and avoid driving or operating potentially dangerous machinery (in the kitchen or workshed as well as at work) if affected.

This side-effect can be a bonus in enabling people to get a good night's sleep, especially for children who lie awake scratching (elixirs as well as tablets are available).

Other temporary side-effects of antihistamines include headache, dry mouth, constipation, blurred vision, gut disturbances and, for some preparations, impotence. Occasionally skin rashes and light-sensitive reactions occur.

Sleeping pills

If severe itching interferes with sleep a doctor may recommend a short course of sleeping pills. While people are rightly wary of becoming dependent on these, as a short-term measure to tide over a miserable, exhausted eczema sufferer until treatments work they can be a lifeline. There is no need to add the misery of uncomfortable, disturbed nights and daytime fatigue, with all its attendant hazards, to the problems you've already got.

Treatment of secondary infections

Although eczema is not contagious or infectious, broken skin (from any cause) becomes more liable to infection. Infection in this way is described as 'secondary infection' because it complicates the primary condition of eczema. The risk is increased by scratching, which may introduce infectious organisms into the skin.

Secondary bacterial infections will be treated with antibiotic creams (sometimes combined with a steroid) or, in severe cases, tablets. If there is a fungal infection (thrush) – as is common with eczema around vulnerable areas such as the ear or groin, with nappy rash and adult seborrhoeic eczema – an antifungal drug will be given.

Although antibiotics are very effective against infected eczema, some doctors feel that they are prescribed too readily. There is a risk of increasing the level of antibiotic resistance in the population so that the drugs cease to be effective against the bacteria most commonly involved.

Case history

Sam's mother brought him to the surgery with eczema on his hands, elbows and knees. She could not stop him from scratching, and the patches were raw and bleeding. While Sam seemed a normal, happy and lively toddler, his mother was clearly worried and exhausted. The family doctor advised using a soap substitute and emollient cream, and prescribed a topical steroid. When this had not helped after a few days, Sam was seen again and the prescription was changed to a steroid-plus-antibiotic cream, which cleared up his skin rapidly. Over the next couple of years, Sam came back every few months with another flare-up, and each time a few days' treatment made it better. The attacks were less and less frequent, and his mother felt the problem was quite manageable. By the time he started school the eczema had almost gone, although he had started having occasional wheezing attacks at night and was prone to colds and runny noses.

Evening primrose oil

Evening primrose oil (EPO) is a traditional herbal remedy for eczema (discussed further in chapter 9) which, following trials, has recently been embraced by conventional medicine and is available on prescription in Britain through the National Health Service.

Many studies have shown that EPO helps eczema, but a few have failed to show any benefit and despite the advance in acceptability some doctors remain sceptical. Still, many do prescribe EPO in childhood eczema, and prescription varieties are suitable for use even in small children (over one year old, at a reduced dose). Special capsules are available which may be snipped open so a child can be given the liquid contents on a teaspoon or smeared on food.

Light treatment

It may seem odd, when some forms of eczema are brought on by sunlight, and when all types may be worsened by heat, that light should also be used as a treatment. Nevertheless doctors have found that sunlight does help many sufferers from atopic eczema (and other skin conditions), and in some cases light therapy may be recommended, usually as an outpatient at the local hospital (though this is more common with psoriasis).

Special lamps are used which give out the rays found in sunlight, and sometimes a tablet (psoralen) is given first to enhance the effect of the light. Repeated treatments may be needed over several weeks. Light treatment is only used in severe cases as the dose must be carefully monitored to avoid side-effects like burning, skin ageing or cataract formation in the eye.

Hyposensitization

The use of hyposensitization – progressively stronger injections of allergens – to desensitize people with specific allergies has been attempted for reactions to pollens, grasses or trees (more commonly for hay fever) and sometimes for food allergies. However this approach has now largely fallen out of favour. Most atopic people are sensitive to many allergens, so it is unlikely to give more than partial relief. More importantly, a severe allergic reaction can be precipitated, and several people (mostly children with asthma) have died as a result. This technique should only be used by specialists for severe, specific allergic reactions, and where facilities for resuscitation are available should a dangerous reaction occur.

Special diets

Many doctors avoid modifying a child's diet, feeling that generally it produces little benefit, is a major inconvenience for the family and makes the child 'different' from others which can cause problems. Obviously if tests for food allergy have proved positive, the doctor will advise avoiding the causes and can help you to plan a diet which does not risk nutritional deficiencies. Some doctors suggest trying a dairy-free diet for atopic infants.

Occasionally if an allergy is found to a common food ingredient which is difficult to avoid a doctor may advise aspirin, or prescribe a drug called *sodium cromoglycate*, to be taken in case of accidental ingestion as these may block some types of reactions (see p. 92).

Assessments of the conventional approach

Unlike some other chronic ailments, conventional medicine has a pretty good understanding of the causes of eczema, does take account of how it is affected by lifestyle, personality and stress levels, and can usually effectively alleviate its symptoms. It cannot, however, offer a cure – and the drug treatments on offer do carry side-effects.

Although they undoubtedly reduce inflammation and relieve symptoms, the heavy reliance on topical steroids for treatment comes in for much criticism from natural therapists who complain, for instance, that:

- Steroids suppress the symptoms without dealing with the cause of the disease
- Steroids suppress the immune system which can lead to a host of other problems
- Symptoms are external signs of inner problems: suppress one and others will appear instead. In an atopic child the lungs are already vulnerable, so steroid creams could increase the risk of asthma later
- Symptoms are the body's way of dealing with disease. Eczema is a defence against foreign or toxic substances, and steroid creams stop the body from cleansing itself.

A conventional response to this might be that steroids are the most effective means of giving relief to the patient, which is what medicine is for, and that doctors are all too well-aware of the potential side-effects and do their best to minimize them and to ensure that patients use them properly.

They could also argue that eczema sufferers are oversensitive to substances normally present in the environment (foods, plants, dust mites and so on), and, broadly speaking, the disease *is* the symptoms produced by this sensitivity. This is quite different from, say, kidney disease, where symptoms stem from a process which actively damages the body, and treatment must avert further damage as well as relieve symptoms. Therefore offering treatment for symptoms is an acceptable approach in the case of eczema since the symptoms *are* the major problem.

CHAPTER 6

The natural therapies and eczema

Introducing the 'gentle alternatives'

Eczema can be resistant to treatment even by the most powerful drugs modern medicine has to offer. Many people have found relief through natural medicine where conventional treatments have failed, or when they have preferred not to expose themselves to strong drugs such as steroids, with all their side-effects. When the time comes to seek help there is a bewildering array of therapies on offer, claiming to be able to help eczema. They include:

- Acupressure (including shiatsu)
- Acupuncture
- Aromatherapy
- Auto-suggestion
- Biofeedback
- Clinical ecology
- Herbal medicine
- Homoeopathy
- Massage, meditation and visualization
- Nutritional medicine
- Reflexology

These therapies will all be discussed in later chapters, as will the all-important matter of finding and choosing a suitable practitioner. But first it is important to understand the beliefs supporting them, for they approach the understanding and treatment of disease from a rather different direction than conventional medicine.

The principles of natural medicine

While the various techniques available are based on a wide range of principles and approaches, they have many characteristics in common. For example:

- They operate 'holistically', which means they take account of the 'whole person' – their mind, body and spirit – as well as their surroundings, lifestyle and relationships.
- They believe good health stems from emotional, mental and physical balance, and that imbalance and disharmony create dis-ease and illness. Often these principles are refined from those of oriental philosophy with its view of a life energy or force (*chi* or *qi*, pronounced 'chee', in China and *prana* in India) and opposing but balanced forces of *yin* and *yang* operating both within the body and throughout the universe.
- They believe the body has a natural ability to heal itself, and the function of treatment is to assist the body's own healing powers.
- Many view symptoms as the body's own attempts to fight disease, and believe that rather than suppressing symptoms treatment should aim to tackle the root cause of the problem.
- The nature of the individual – their emotions, personality, reactions and circumstances – is seen as at least as important in determining therapy as the disease or symptoms themselves. Therefore two people with the same condition will not necessarily receive the same treatment.

What to expect when you see a natural therapist

The above principles lead to several differences in approach from those you may be used to with a family doctor. For example:

- Consultations usually take much longer (at least an hour)
- You are likely to be asked a wide range of questions about yourself, your emotions, your job, family, relationships and social life, what you eat and drink, your sleeping and relaxation habits
- Therapy is likely to involve advice about your lifestyle (diet, exercise, sleep, emotions and so on) as well as any specific treatments like pills or massage
- Therapy will not necessarily be directed only at the problem you came with, but may encompass any aspects the therapist feels are out of balance
- Treatments may take longer to work because they attempt to get to the roots of a problem rather than offering rapid symptom relief
- They thus often require more patience, time and effort, and a greater commitment to change. You will generally be expected to take responsibility for your own health and to be actively involved in the healing process

Why people turn to natural medicine

Most people turn to natural therapists after years, sometimes decades, of conventional treatment has failed. In one survey of patients visiting a British natural health centre most had long-standing problems (an average of nine years), almost all had seen their family doctor (and many a specialist) first. Most found their doctor helpful and understanding but conventional medicine had not been able to solve their problems. Most patients felt they had received 'satisfactory' treatment, yet stated that its failure was the reason for seeking other help. Allergic symptoms such as eczema, asthma, urticaria and rhinitis were the second most common reason for attending.

Does it work?

In the same survey nearly two-thirds of people said they had experienced some improvement with natural treatments, and those who believed that the methods worked were more likely to benefit. (It may be that nature therapies have more to offer for the sort of long-term ailments often termed 'diseases of civilization', like allergies, migraine, rheumatism, stress and depression, whereas orthodox medicine is very good at dealing with acute or life-threatening illnesses, like infections, cancer or acute appendicitis.)

A UK survey of members of the public in the mid-1980s showed that although relatively few people had tried natural treatments, most of those who had were satisfied with the results.

	Satisfied (%)	Dissatisfied (%)
Herbal medicine	73	18
Vitamin therapy	65	12
Osteopathy	73	14
Massage	82	9
Homoeopathy	66	16
Meditation/relaxation	83	12
Acupuncture	50	47
Chiropractic	68	19
Healing	68	16
Hypnotherapy	43	50
Psychotherapy	75	12

What do doctors think of it?

The attitude of doctors to natural medicine ranges from
the few who still dismiss all non-conventional approaches out of hand as 'fringe' or worse, to the increasing
numbers who are adding training in techniques such as
homoeopathy, acupuncture, hypnosis and herbal medicine to their conventional qualifications.

In the middle are the majority of doctors who are
often more broad-minded about natural medicine than
their patients may imagine. Some may feel vaguely
bemused or sceptical, but most are at least interested
and usually prepared to concede that, in general, natural
therapies do no harm.

The most common reservations about natural medicine are:

- The lack of formal evaluation (research) of many treatments
- How they work, or are supposed to work, often cannot
  be explained in conventional scientific terms
- There is (at present) little regulation of most practitioners and few safeguards for patients against the occasional unscrupulous or unethical therapist
- Serious diseases may be missed or mis-diagnosed
- A few practitioners advise patients to abandon orthodox treatment altogether, which can be dangerous in
  life-threatening conditions.

Some natural methods are difficult to test in the sort of
formal trials which conventional medicines undergo.
Since prescriptions do not follow the conventional one-
symptom/one-drug approach they often differ for two
people with the 'same' condition or symptoms, and
involve multiple approaches which may be impossible
to separate. Nevertheless many practitioners are con-
ducting formal studies of their therapies, and an impres-

sive body of evidence is accumulating for many treatments.

The accustomed rivalry between conventional and natural medicine is gradually lessening, and increasingly conventional doctors are offering natural (which they mostly prefer to call 'complementary') treatments themselves or are prepared to refer their patients to reputable local practitioners.

In Britain, for example, where surveys have shown that nearly 40% of doctors have had some training in unconventional approaches (and some 2000 are now qualified in homoeopathy), one in four are happy to refer patients to a natural therapist. Such a combined approach is an excellent safeguard for patients and a hopeful sign for the medicine of the next century, which must expect to deal with many more chronic degenerative diseases in an ageing population.

How do natural therapies treat eczema?

Natural therapists tend to see eczema as a reflection of many individual factors. For example, they may view the frequency or severity of eczema attacks as representing the internal state of health, energy balance or psychological stability of the individual. Most believe that exposure to an irritant or allergy-provoking substance is only part of the story, and general health determines how the individual responds.

What you eat, how much exercise you take, whether you smoke or drink to excess, how much stress you are under at work and the state of your marriage may all be relevant to how they approach the problem. For a child, family tension, the relationship between parents, how well brothers and sisters get on, poor home circumstances, bullying, poor performance or unhappiness at school could all influence the sensitivity of the skin.

As well as sometimes helping skin symptoms directly, treatment may be directed towards:

- Counteracting psychological trauma
- Combatting stress
- Encouraging a healthy lifestyle
- Stimulating the elimination of toxins from the body
- Promoting healthy skin defence mechanisms
- Realigning the body's energy balance
- Encouraging a harmonious attitude to life, work and relationships.

Assessing the options

In deciding between various forms of therapy, conventional or natural, remember there is nothing to stop you trying different approaches (especially when nothing seems to be working), or picking the parts you like from different systems. However, you do need to give each method a fair trial, and make sure that they do not clash with each other. A conventional doctor would want to know about natural treatment in case it affects the drugs you are taking. Similarly, a homoeopath will almost certainly have a different approach for someone who has already used, say, steroid creams for their eczema, and it makes sense to tell whatever practitioner you see what else you have already tried.

In the following chapters the approaches of the various natural treatments are discussed, along with the evidence that they can help the symptoms of eczema and reduce the frequency and severity of attacks.

For how to find and choose a natural therapist see chapter 10.

CHAPTER 7

Treating your mind and emotions

Therapies for how you think and feel

Eczema, like all skin diseases, affects more than the skin. Unlike, say, kidney disease, where the sufferer can generally choose who to tell and when, skin is public property. It is also an intimate organ, crucial to our feeling senses and vital to our emotional well-being: we need to feel 'at home' within it and receptive to hugs through it.

As noted in chapter one, eczema may have dire consequences for an individual's self-confidence, work, hobbies, social life and relationships. Difficult-to-follow avoidance and treatment regimes can lead to added pressure and guilt over lapses, especially if the condition recurs. It is hardly surprising if sufferers at times feel angry, miserable or despairing. Almost all forms of therapy recognize that emotional tension can make eczema worse, so clearly people with eczema can find themselves locked in a vicious spiral of skin and emotional problems.

None of this means that eczema is 'all in the mind' or that symptoms are unreal. The more medical science looks into the mind-body link, the more evidence it finds that mind and body are inextricably interlinked, and the mind has a profound effect on almost every disease investigated. Most ancient civilizations regarded mind, body and spirit as parts of the same whole; it is only recently that Western cultures have considered them in isolation.

Personality and illness.

Doctors recognize that aggressive, ambitious, driven people, the so-called 'type A personality' of a typical high-flyer, are more coronary-prone than laid-back 'type B' people. This well-known example is interesting because it can be partly explained by known biological responses to stress, and because type A people can be trained to have a more type B attitude, and so reduce their risk of heart attacks.

However other links with personality, such as the so-called cancer-prone personality (over-concerned with fulfilling others' needs while repressing their own desires, anger and resentment), are hotly disputed. So is the theory that people with eczema are guilt-ridden worriers who suppress their emotions and are hypersensitive in an emotional sense, as well as on their skin.

But it does neatly fit with psychologist Carl Jung's idea that illness has a symbolic meaning – someone with unexplained nausea might be 'sick of it all', painful shoulders might mean carrying too great a burden unsupported. Could someone with skin disease be irritated by their life circumstances, or itching to get away from something?

On the other hand, that could be bunkum. Humans may have a peculiar need to attribute illness which cannot be scientifically explained to psychological factors. People with tuberculosis were seen as having a particular, susceptible personality, until the tuberculosis bacterium was discovered. If people with eczema are extra sensitive to stress, that could well be a consequence rather than a cause of their eczema, or it could be because children with eczema tend to be intelligent, which often goes with 'sensitivity'.

There could be purely mechanical links – people who 'suppress' their feelings about the disease are less likely to care for their skin, while those who are extra 'sensitive' to it may continually pour irritant creams on their skin.

The explanation perhaps matters less than the facts that surveys have shown that one-third or more of skin patients are in a state of psychological distress, and the workings of the mind indisputably affect our bodily state (and vice-versa).

The psychology of the body

Think, for instance, of the way you might react to a sudden explosion, nearby but not so close as to injure you. Chances are your heart would pound, and you might go white, tremble or even faint. That is a perfectly understandable instance of a 'psychological' reaction (fear) influencing the body.

Our bodies are geared by millions of years of evolution to react to stress physically, the classic 'fight-or-flight' reaction necessary for dealing with prehistoric life, when delaying to think could end in being eaten. The trouble is that our bodies still run that way, even though wild beasts are not the problem in most modern offices, troubled marriages, crowded tube trains or high-pressure meetings.

Evidence for the influence of mind on body

- Just thinking about sucking a lemon stimulates saliva flow
- Many people's blood pressure rises when a doctor takes it rather than someone else ('white coat hypertension')
- Serious sporting injuries may go unnoticed until the final whistle, when the player stops concentrating on the game
- People behave as if drunk if they believe they are

drinking alcohol even when they are given a no-alcohol fake
- Emotions affect the immune system
- Among breast cancer patients, those who react with fighting spirit do better than those who passively submit to fate
- People seem able to 'put off' dying until after events or celebrations which are important to them
- Patients' expectations of the effectiveness of treatment influence the outcome

The placebo effect

The placebo effect is what happens when someone who believes that an inert 'sugar pill' contains an active drug reacts as if they had taken the drug itself. It is much maligned (especially when used scornfully as an explanation for the workings of natural therapies), yet it is an exceptionally powerful but under-used medical tool.

For instance, one study showed that a dose of morphine was effective in relieving pain in about 70 per cent of subjects tested. But when given a placebo they believed to be morphine, 35 per cent reported a pain-killing effect. This implies that up to half of the effect of morphine, one of the most powerful drugs available in medicine, may be attributable to the mind. One great medical teacher was famous for saying that we should not underestimate the placebo effect of the drug 'doctor'. The confidence with which a doctor hands out a medicine can influence its efficacy (hence the importance of a good 'bedside manner'). This means that if you approach novel treatments, lifestyle changes or stress management techniques with a positive attitude they are more likely to help (and similarly if you don't, they won't).

Who would 'want' to be ill?

If the mind can help recovery it can also hinder it. Some people resist the idea that stress is a factor in their illness, and studies have shown that they tend to have some reason (often unconscious) to hang onto their problem, despite its discomforts. It has definite benefits, known as secondary gain, such as gaining attention from a spouse, sympathy from friends, or enabling them to avoid certain activities. Others may have such painful underlying emotions that they cannot bear to confront them: for example, someone in a bad marriage may not wish to face the possibility that they should leave.

Also eczema can become overwhelmingly important in someone's life. It is irritating and unsightly, and can affect every aspect of daily living, so is difficult to forget. Tracking down the cause can involve months of detective work, followed by major alterations to well-ingrained habits. Sufferers may be continually explaining why their work is restricted and they cannot stroke someone's pet, help with domestic chores or eat food at a dinner party. A few people (not many, but some) become so wrapped-up in their condition that they become obsessive and boring about it.

Expectations affect disease and its treatment, and some types of eczema (food intolerance, in particular) can become a 'learned response', in which the person somehow creates the symptoms he or she believes will result from a particular circumstance. Eczema should not come to dominate your life, and that of those around you, and if it seems to be doing so, seek help.

Making stress work for you

Stress makes us tense and irritable. In the long term it can raise our blood pressure and increase our susceptibility to illness. Reducing their level of stress helps many people to avoid flare-ups of eczema. The brain and the skin develop from the same cells in the embryo. The autonomic nervous system, the part involved in stress and largely outside conscious control, also regulates flushing, sweating and hair erection in the skin. It may be that prolonged over-stimulation of these nerves in stress reactions leads to various skin diseases and symptoms. Itching in particular may be a stress-related response.

But not all stress is bad. Stress is just a form of arousal, and without arousal there is no incentive to do anything – we are least stressed (nightmares excepted) when asleep or comatose. There is an optimum level of arousal, up to which our performance is enhanced, and beyond which we become so aroused that instead of being alert and attentive we fall over the edge into anxiety and reduced performance. If we operate consistently above our threshold level of stress, we run a high risk of stress-related illness. The key is to spot when we approach the critical threshold, and learn to stay on the healthy side of the curve.

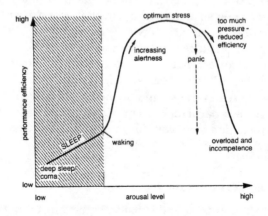

Fig. 3 'Good' and 'bad' stress

Case histories

Jenny had severe eczema as a child, which cleared up when she was about ten but occasionally flared up in small patches. When she was 28 she was offered a promotion to chief buyer of the fashion-chain she worked for, a job she thought she wanted although it meant moving some 200 miles away. Then her eczema flared up badly, and she started dreading going to work because her hands seemed so unsightly. She became very distressed and had difficulty sleeping, so her GP referred her to a psychologist. She realized she did not want to move, turned down the promotion, and her eczema receded again.

Henry is a bachelor aged 40 who still lives with his mother and has suffered from eczema all his life. When his mother had to go into hospital for an extended stay, his skin cleared up. His specialist pointed out that maybe he disliked living with his mother, but he refused point-blank to consider finding a home of his own. When his mother was discharged, his eczema came back.

Martine is 12 and has had eczema since she was a toddler. It started with the birth of a younger brother, and gets worse whenever there is tension in the family. Her parents feel guilty, and always give her loads of attention and special treats whenever her skin is bad. Her latest skin specialist has recommended a careful routine of skin care and a new type of cream which seems to work, but Martine keeps playing with her brother's pet gerbil even though she knows it makes her skin flare up.

Is your eczema related to emotions?

The more yes answers you give to the questions below, the more likely it is that psychological factors are operating:

- Do you know that stress makes the symptoms worse?
- Are you generally a worrier or anxious about everyday events?
- Are you easily upset but prefer not to show it?
- Do you generally react to stress with physical symptoms – flushing, pounding heart beat, rapid breathing, feeling sick or butterflies in the stomach?
- Do you talk about your eczema regularly to people outside your immediate family and friends?
- Do you sometimes feel you overreact to your symptoms?
- If your skin improves, are you the last to notice?
- Do you do things which you know make your skin worse – handle irritants, eat the wrong foods, scratch, take hot baths?
- Do you often fail to take prescribed treatments, or not follow the instructions properly?
- Do you blame other people for making your skin flare up?
- If you are offered a new treatment, do you assume it will not work?

In a child

- Does the child's eczema get worse when you are tense, or after family quarrels?
- Did it start or does it flare up at crisis points – new members of the family, changing schools, taking exams?
- Do you feel especially guilty, tense or unhappy about the child's skin?
- Do you make a fuss about the child's skin, attempt to cover up, or discuss it with others in front of the child?
- Do you think of, or refer to, the child as being 'sensitive' or delicate?

How to help yourself

Learning to relax can mean anything from a soak in a hot bath to taking 30 seconds out to take a deep breath in the middle of a stressed morning, but is most likely to be effective if done regularly, consciously and without guilt. Recognize it takes practice, so you will not instantly be able to handle high stress situations with total calmness, you need to build up your resistance gradually.

Our psychological state is affected by almost every aspect of life: our diet, how much exercise we take, the air we breathe, what we do and who we live with, where and how we live, why we live. One of the greatest keys to good health and happiness is having a purpose in life, a goal outside ourselves. This is one of the great benefits of religion, but you don't have to be religious to be involved in something. Good health means treating our bodies with respect, feeding our minds as much as our stomachs, developing our interests and keeping setbacks in proportion.

Some general tips are:

- Get out of doors as much as possible. People who work indoors under artificial lights may be deprived of healthy light, which can lead to depression, and skin needs fresh air as much as the lungs
- Wear natural fabrics which allow the skin to breathe
- Take regular exercise
- Walk tall – posture is important to mental state, and going around with hunched shoulders, or slumping when sitting, will make you feel low
- Eat a healthy diet, avoid additives and pollutants wherever possible
- Get enough sleep and rest
- Try to keep harmonious relationships with those closest to you

- Cultivate a purpose in life – work, hobby, art, religion, it doesn't matter (except beware focusing too much on your children: one day they have to live a life of their own)
- Develop a fulfilling social life
- Get involved in neighbourhood activities so you feel integrated with your community and valued by others
- Stay in touch with nature
- Try to keep a healthy level of reality in your life, don't experience it all second-hand through TV and videos. If you feel down, giving up newspapers and TV news bulletins (which are generally depressing) for a month can have a remarkably uplifting effect
- Take time off, unplug the telephone when you don't want to be disturbed, learn to say no to others' demands (assertiveness training can help if this is difficult)

There are numerous de-stressing techniques which you can try yourself at home:

Progressive muscular relaxation

People often carry their bodies in a state of perpetual tension, especially around the shoulders, neck and jaw muscles, and this exercise helps to release it. It involves first tensing then relaxing muscle groups, working up the body from the toes to the head. Lie comfortably on your back in a quiet room where you will not be disturbed. Clench the toes of one foot hard, then relax them. Tighten then relax the muscles of your ankle, calf, knees, thighs and hips, then repeat the whole process with your other leg. Flow up the body doing the same, including the muscles at the top of your scalp, round your eyes and around your jaw.

If any part of your body feels as if it is tensing up

again, squeeze and relax once more. Try to stay in a relaxed state for at least ten minutes, and do the exercise daily if you can. It can be used alongside visualization or meditation.

Positive affirmations/Auto-suggestion

These are repeated positive messages that you say to yourself or out loud. The classic is "every day in every way I am getting better and better", but you can invent your own. Repeat them at least 25 times, ideally in the morning when you wake up and at night just before you go to sleep, when the subconscious is most receptive. They encourage a positive outlook and, perhaps more importantly, silence for a while the nagging, critical ticker-tape which many people have running as background in their heads throughout the day. Affirmation is just a modern word for auto-suggestion, a form of self-hypnosis claimed to reduce stress, alleviate symptoms and help clear skin-rashes:

- Keep the messages short and, if possible, rhythmic
- Avoid negative words (the subconscious does not register them, so you may get the opposite effect to the one intended): "I want clean healthy lungs" rather than "I do not want a cigarette"
- Keep in the present (even if your aim has not yet come true): "I am getting better", not "I will get better"
- Stay personal: it's no use wishing someone else (or the universe) would change
- Use visualization as well to enhance the effect.

Visualization

The imagination has a powerful effect on the body, and imagining your body as successful in fighting disease can help in overcoming it. Although early claims of dramatic cures in conditions such as cancer have not been sustained, visualization can have great psychological benefits, especially in stress reduction, and also by visualizing a positive outcome to forthcoming events or goals, such as 'seeing' yourself weighing ten pounds less.

Follow the instructions for progressive muscular relaxation then begin to imagine a beautiful scene – it could be a favourite holiday place you know, or somewhere totally imaginary. It is your place, with no tensions, no one to worry you. Look around in your mind's eye, see every detail, try to capture other senses: smells, sounds, the feel of grass on your bare feet. If you want to try some self-healing, you could imagine the warmth of the sun healing your skin, or see red patches just floating off as you let go of the problem. Once you become adept at such visualizations, you can use them as a rapid first aid almost anywhere: if you suddenly feel the urge to scratch, for instance, you can try imagining the itch as an ugly little leprechaun dancing on your skin, then blow him off and see him floating away to the far end of the room.

Meditation

Meditation clears the mind of all the mental rattles and toxins which accumulate day by day. It need involve no oriental mysticism, and can easily be learned at home. It takes 10 or 20 minutes once or twice a day (although as one harrassed mother said, "if I had twenty minutes twice a day to myself to meditate, I wouldn't be so stressed as to need to").

Meditation has been used in hospitals to help patients reduce high blood pressure without drugs. It produces measurable changes in brain-waves, muscular tension, circulation and breathing patterns. Many people with stress-related eczema find it helps enormously.

Choose a quiet room, sit comfortably with your legs uncrossed and your hands resting loosely on your lap, eyes open or closed as you prefer, breathing in through your nose if possible. The aim is to keep your mind clear of all arousing thoughts, and the simplest way to do this is to replace them with something else. There are several options, which can be combined:

- A mantra – any short word, repeated over and over. It could be a meaningless sound, a non-stimulating word like 'the', or a calming one like 'peace'.
- Following the breath – without making any effort to alter its rhythm and flow imagine the air travelling in through your nose, down into your lungs, up and out again. After a while make your breaths 'diaphragmatic' by moving your abdomen rather than your chest, and exhale completely and for at least as long as you inhaled on each breath.
- Focusing on an object, either real (for example, a candle) or imaginary (a large red circle). Look at its edges, sweep your eyes round and inside it, imagine its feel or smell, concentrate on it and nothing else.

Don't worry if thoughts intrude (many people are surprised by how short a time they can last before they do – it gets longer with practice), just push them away and carry on. You may find that playing a soothing tape (without words), or scenting the room with an aromatherapy fragrance, aids the sense of calm.

SEEKING HELP

Massage Massage is deliciously sensual and relaxing whether done at home with a partner to relieve stress and tension, or professionally, perhaps in conjunction with treatments such as aromatherapy.

Aromatherapy Aromatherapy uses essential oils of aromatic plants, usually diluted in a base oil, such as almond, jojoba or even extra virgin olive oil (which itself soothes inflamed skin), to enhance massage or as a component of beauty treatments. It is offered in many health farms, beauty salons and natural treatment centres, and practitioners say that it helps maintain health, energy and vitality, and aids the body's powers of self-healing for minor ailments.

Apart from helping relaxation and controlling the stress which can make eczematous reactions worse, practitioners say the skin can respond directly to oils concentrated from the following:

- *Camomile* – anti-inflammatory and sedative, helpful for eczema triggered by anxiety, or itching interfering with sleep
- *Lavender* – soothes sore skin, useful for nervous tension
- *Cedarwood* – helps both skin and respiratory tract
- *Juniper berries* – help weeping skin to heal

Note cedarwood and juniper oils should never be used during pregnancy.

- *Patchouli* and *calendula* - help dry or cracked skin
- *Sandalwood, hyssop, geranium* and *fennel* – assist skin healing.

It is a good idea to visit a practitioner first to see which oils you like before buying for home use as they are quite expensive, and some people are allergic to the oils themselves. Never use aromatherapy for a baby or small child without expert guidance, and be extremely cautious in pregnancy. Essential oils can be powerful and some are potentially toxic. They should always be diluted according to the recommendations of a comprehensive guide (see Appendix B), and never be taken by mouth except under the guidance of a qualified aromatherapist.

Flower Remedies Flower essences are remedies for stress and emotional imbalance, first devised by a homoeopathic physician, Dr Edward Bach (pronounced 'batch'). They were initially prepared homoeopathically (see p. 114), and later by soaking petals in sunlight or boiling them, which he believed to imbue the solution with the healing life energy of the flower.

Many natural practitioners, especially herbalists, aromatherapists and health and beauty clinics, incorporate flower remedies into their practice, and they can also be bought from many healthfood and herbal suppliers (dilute before use).

As with homoeopathic remedies, they are prescribed according to personality but some are commonly used for skin-complaints:

- *Crab apple* – especially for those who feel self-conscious or ugly about their skin
- *Clematis* and *mimulus* - for hypersensitive skin
- *Impatiens* – if irritable because of itching or self-consciousness
- *'Rescue Remedy'* cream – rub on affected areas.

Yoga This is based on ancient Indian philosophy which views body energy (see p. 94) as concentrated in *chakras*, invisible centres of different colours and qualities running from the base of the spine to the top of the head. Energy balance is restored and flow realigned by various postural and breathing exercises, meditation and diet. Yoga has been shown to help reduce high blood pressure and control asthma as well as relieving stress. Self-teaching manuals are available, but it is best to go to classes to learn yoga, which can then be practised at home. It is an excellent, gentle way to relax and re-tone the body and can help stress-related eczema.

Autogenic training This is a form of autosuggestion involving a set of phrases and exercises to produce specific bodily sensations, which needs to be taught (usually as a group). It can be used for relaxation, general health or treatment of various conditions such as migraine, anxiety and high blood pressure.

Biofeedback   Biofeedback machines measure changes such as blood pressure, skin temperature and muscle tension. They demonstrate that relaxation, meditation and yoga lower blood pressure, and are used in lie-detector tests (based on alterations of the skin under stress). They can show people how to alter functions not normally thought to be under conscious control, and are useful in reducing anxiety and blood pressure, improving poor circulation, alleviating migraine, asthma and tics, treating addictions and aborting panic attacks. Devices vary from simple meters showing a scale read-out to modern versions using video game techniques.

Colour therapy   This is a relatively new therapy (although many of its practitioners say colour has been used for healing since the days of ancient Egypt). It does not take much imagination to realize that a person suffering from stress will be better off in a room painted a tranquil shade of blue than one with lurid orange and purple stripes. But there are in fact much more subtle effects which are increasingly used in social psychology. For example:

- Blues and greens have a calming effect which may help in waiting rooms and hospitals
- Certain shades of pink reduce agitation and aggression, and when used in police cells can help calm violent criminals
- Bright reds and oranges make people eat faster in restaurants
- Deep red colours can produce a womb-like security which may be useful for mental patients.

Hypnotherapy Hypnosis is an altered state of consciousness in which the mind becomes more receptive to suggestions. It gained a bad reputation through its use in stage-shows and still worries many people, even though it is now practised increasingly by doctors and psychologists and is widely used in childbirth and dentistry.

It can be highly effective in stress-related illnesses and skin diseases, making warts disappear, relieving *urticaria* and altering contact sensitivities. In experiments, people under hypnosis may react to something they believe is an irritant or allergen, even if it is not. Conversely, they may be able to handle true irritants without harm if told they are non-toxic.

Practitioners claim that they can cure most people with stress-related eczema (assuming they are suitable for hypnosis) in two or three sessions. Many hypnotherapists teach people techniques of self-hypnosis to use between and after treatment sessions. The experience of hypnosis should not be at all scary as it is really a form of deep relaxation, like meditation or 'talking to yourself on the inside' – but choose a reputable practitioner.

Psychological treatments Some form of psychological therapy may be useful when there is a strong emotional element to eczema, especially in adults who have had skin problems since childhood, and who feel generally unhappy with their lives.

There is a bewildering variety of therapies available, and the best bet is either to go by personal recommendation or to spend some time reading about the different approaches to see which, if any, might suit you. Be aware, too, of the potential pitfalls: there is a risk of becoming too dependent on the therapist and on therapy itself. It is important not to let therapy become the dominant force in your life without making effective changes outside the consulting room. There is an increasing 'anti-therapy' movement, especially in the USA, which holds that therapy does not work and may be positively harmful.

Most private therapy is expensive – psycho-analysis particularly so as it usually takes several sessions a week over months or years, and so requires a strong commitment. Some newer therapies were developed to achieve change in a shorter time, and many academic and private institutions run short courses and workshops for people to sample the techniques.

CHAPTER 8

Food and diet treatments

How what you eat can help your skin

Many cases of atopic eczema may be due to a specific food sensitivity. People who are undernourished or have specific vitamin deficiencies also become more prone to skin disease. So it makes sense that eating a healthy diet can strengthen the skin and reduce sensitivity generally, so can help with contact reactions as well as specific food-allergies.

Eating tips to help your skin

- Eat fewer animal fats
- Eat more fresh fruit and vegetables
- Avoid heavily processed and 'junk' foods
- Cut down on sugar and alcohol
- Increase consumption of vegetable oils and oily fish
- Take regular supplements of
    Evening primrose oil (see p. 109)
    Fish oils
    Vitamins A, B and E
    Zinc, selenium and magnesium.

It is often said that people eating a typical 'western' diet are overfed but undernourished. They eat too much of the wrong kinds of foods – animal fats, salt, sugar, processed foods, fast foods and junk food. In the process they take in pesticides, preservatives and colouring

additives – all of which are increasingly recognized as
potentially harmful – and they do not get enough fresh
fruit and vegetables or fibre. It is perhaps because the
balance of our diet is so 'unnatural' that people are
becoming more prone to food-related diseases and allergies.

Dairy products

Many practitioners in both natural and, increasingly,
conventional medicine believe food allergies are very
important in atopic eczema, with dairy products particularly to blame such as eggs, milk, butter, cheese,
yoghurt, cream, and products containing skimmed-milk
powder or whey. Many will regard a child with eczema
as allergic to eggs or milk until proved otherwise.

Nutritionists often say that cows' milk is unsuitable
food for humans since it is linked with lactose (milk
sugar) intolerance, heart disease and over-production of
catarrh and mucus (as traditional Indian *Ayurvedic* practitioners believe also). It has been linked, too, with
hyperactivity, joint and blood diseases, asthma, hay
fever and even cot deaths.

Many babies develop eczema as they are weaned
from breast milk, which is another good reason to breast-
feed for as long as possible. Some nutritionists advise
delaying the introduction of dairy foods until the child is
at least six months and preferably one or even two years
old. There are several substitute milk products designed
for infants, although some unfortunate babies are also
allergic to soya, the most common alternative source.

Even breast-fed babies may, if very sensitive, develop
reactions to food items in their mothers' milk. Cows'
milk and egg proteins, like other allergens, may come
out in breast milk, or it may be the mother's own antibodies to these items – often the mother in such cases is
sensitive too. Frequently if a breast-feeding mother

avoids dairy products herself the child's eczema improves (and this tactic also helps about one in three babies with infant colic).

Tracking food intolerance

If you suspect a food reaction but the cause is not obvious, keeping a food diary may help to spot links with what you eat. As well as dairy products, other common culprits in atopic eczema include fish, wheat, sugar, food additives, citrus fruits, tomatoes and yeast-containing foods.

If the cause of a food reaction can be pinpointed (about one-third of cases), eczema often clears within a matter of days when it is removed from the diet, although for some foods including dairy products it may take up to three weeks or more before any improvement is seen. It is therefore important to remove only one food or food group at a time to avoid nutritional deficiencies.

You can confirm a food intolerance by avoiding it for a month or so after the eczema has cleared, then including it in the diet again to see if symptoms reappear. Some people are never able to tolerate that particular food again, but many can re-introduce it after a few months. The longer the period of avoidance the more chance that sensitivity will have lessened.

Avoidance does not always get rid of symptoms entirely as many people are sensitive to several allergens, but they are usually substantially reduced. The fact that a particular food is not always linked with eczema does not rule it out as a possible cause because stress can sometimes trigger a reaction to foods you may be susceptible to but normally able to tolerate.

While many patients can experiment for themselves by eliminating common allergens, it is vital not to restrict the diet too much. Unless you have rapid success with simple measures it is sensible to consult a qualified practitioner, and always seek professional advice before making long-term changes to a child's diet.

Seeking help

Many conventional and most natural therapists offer nutritional advice either as the major treatment or as an adjunct to their own particular approach to eczema. Therapies which rely heavily on dietary methods to deal with eczema include:
• Nutritional medicine
• Clinical ecology
• Naturopathy
• Biochemic tissue salts
• Ayurvedic medicine.

Special diets

If the source of eczema cannot readily be identified by keeping a food diary, a practitioner may supervise an 'elimination diet' (sometimes also called an 'exclusion diet': see p. 46-7) to try to pin-point causes. There are several varieties:
• Five-day fast (bottled spring water only) – should only be undertaken supervised by a doctor, dietician or nutritionist
• Lamb and pears diet (see p. 46)
• Modified elimination diets – various, for adults, children and particular conditions.
Some children get eczema in response to more than one food, and many 'atopics' have other food allergies too (for instance, causing infant colic, sleep disturbances, hyperactivity or asthma), so this may help to identify the source of other problems. In adult atopic eczema an elimination diet can sometimes pin-point a food responsible for years of misery.

Special diagnostic techniques

The following few specialist diagnostic techniques are commonly employed by various natural therapists and by some doctors interested in nutritional approaches:

Iridology   This claims to detect internal disorders (including those behind eczema) in the patterns of the iris of the eye using a torch and magnifying glass or photography with special equipment. But there is little or no conclusive evidence for its claims and most doctors are sceptical.

Hair analysis   This is often used to assess nutritional deficiencies and diagnose allergies. A lock of hair is taken from the neckline at the back of the scalp (where it grows fastest), and sent off to a laboratory. Hair protein (*keratin*) absorbs minerals so analysis can spot poisons like aluminium or lead, said to accumulate in a few food intolerant people, and show deficiencies or overload of vital elements like calcium, magnesium or copper. Conventional opinion is divided but some doctors do use hair analysis as an extra diagnostic tool.

Kinesiology   This is a diagnostic system based on energy flow through the body (see p. 99). It is often used to identify food allergies or nutritional imbalances which are said to cause weakness of specific muscles. The strength of major muscle groups is tested by holding a limb (usually an arm) steady against gentle pressure. The limb is then re-tested while the patient holds particular substances in the hand or, for foods, between the lips. Loss of strength suggests allergy, an increase may reveal deficiency states. Again, most conventional practitioners are sceptical although a few use the technique themselves. There is little research to back up the value of kinesiology in diagnosis but there is no doubt that many people do experience quite dramatic differences in muscle-power during testing.

Some nutritionists will recommend a rotation diet, in which foods are rotated over a period of four to seven days so that the same food is not eaten twice in this period. This both encourages tolerance of foods to which the patient was formerly sensitive and, in patients who react to components of many staple foods, reduces the risk of developing further sensitivities because other foods are being eaten in greater quantities.

Nutritional medicine

Many well-conducted studies have pointed to the effectiveness of nutritional medicine in a wide range of conditions, especially the kind of long-term illnesses often described as 'diseases of civilization' (and perhaps of Western foods), such as migraine, arthritis, irritable bowel syndrome, depression, asthma and eczema.

Various forms of elimination or rotation diet may be suggested, and sometimes the special diagnostic tests and desensitization programmes used in clinical ecology (see below). Specific remedies which may be advised for eczema include:

- Calcium supplements (some people with allergies are deficient)
- Magnesium and vitamin B6 for women whose eczema seems worse before a period
- Women on the Pill may be recommended to stop taking it to see if this makes any difference
- Some people with eczema have been found to have a deficiency of stomach acids, which can be uncovered by a simple test, and treated by replacement supplements and B vitamins
- Raw juice treatment (carrot, beetroot, cucumber and celery)
- Propolis cream or capsules (for dry eczema only)

- Honey may help stress-related eczema (a teaspoonful 4-6 times daily) and, if taken regularly early in the year, may reduce later sensitivity to pollen in hay fever (use local honey to give the right mix of pollens for your area)
- Additive avoidance, especially benzoates (E210-219), linked with skin problems, asthma and hay fever
- A teaspoon of baking soda in water may help to reduce food allergic reactions after accidental eating.

Clinical ecology

Clinical ecology is a branch of conventional medicine whose approach to food reactions is more akin to that of some natural techniques, and which in some respects overlaps with nutritional medicine. It holds that modern lifestyles are far removed from the 'primitive' conditions to which humans are biologically tuned.

Many influences, from lead in water pipes, pesticides and industrial pollution contaminating our crops and atmosphere, to additives in our foods and the salt and sugar we pour on them, can be regarded as potentially toxic, and their spread in the environment has far outpaced human ability to adapt. Food and chemical sensitivity are therefore becoming increasingly common, and are estimated to affect 10-30 per cent of people in Western countries.

An ecological approach may help all kinds of 'modern' ailments such as obesity, asthma, eczema, hay fever, migraine, arthritis and inflammatory bowel disease. A range of symptoms such as depression, anxiety, chronic fatigue or insomnia which a conventional doctor might put down to stress are seen by the ecologist as possible signs of food or chemical sensitivity. The reason that some people develop such sensitivities when others do not is little understood, but suggestions include hereditary tendencies, abnormal gut bacteria, exposure to pesticides and other toxic chemicals, viral infections, nutritional deficiencies and electrical pollution.

'Sensitivity' may not be the same as a full-blown allergic response with antibody production. It could, for instance, be due to abnormal gut sensitivity or enzyme deficiencies so that foods are not fully broken down and metabolized properly. Hence the diseases which result often cannot be defined or tested-for in purely allergic terms (although because people often refer to them as allergies some immunity experts scoff at clinical ecology). Nevertheless, many patients respond when treated as if they were allergic.

A particularly important concept is that of 'masked sensitivity'. Symptoms do not necessarily appear at once (another confusion for conventional doctors), and may be due to multiple sensitivities which gradually overwhelm the body's capacity to adapt. One sensitivity makes it more likely that others will develop as the body is already weakened. Masked sensitivities may accumulate to cause a state of chronic ill-health, or appear as disease when something else, such as stress, is added on top. Furthermore, in some cases the body's attempts to adapt to a substance to which it is sensitive can lead to addiction – in much the same way that an alcoholic addicted to drink has withdrawal symptoms when he suddenly stops even though the alcohol is poisoning his body.

Where conventional medicine generally sees symptoms as a direct consequence of an underlying disease, clinical ecologists see sensitivity as the underlying problem which may cause a variety of symptoms even within the same individual. A child with sensitivity to cows' milk could, for example, progress from infant colic to eczema to asthma and hay fever, perhaps with attacks of catarrh and ear infections thrown in.

Eczema is seen as an inherited susceptibility with precipitating factors including climate, irritants, stress and allergies, especially to food but also to common allergens like house dust mite, and to chemicals, even those present in tap water. Some children may have a fungal infection within the intestine (*candidiasis*), which ecologists believe weakens the lining and promotes food intolerance.

Several specialized tests (as well as those described above) may be used to identify allergies and sensitivities. Their results are heavily dependent on the skill and experience of the practitioner, but some claim success in 80 per cent of patients (see box on page 90).

In clinical ecology, dealing with responsible external factors is a matter of adjusting lifestyle and habits, so responsibility for treatment is placed firmly in the hands of the patient.

For food sensitivities, particularly if masked, a curious sequence emerges where if a patient avoids the incriminated food for a week or so (during which there may be a variety of withdrawal symptoms including craving the food in question) eating that food at any time over the next few weeks will produce a more severe response than before (known as 'hypersensitivity'). After a couple of months' avoidance, in many people the same food may be tolerated provided it is not eaten too often (or masked sensitivity can again develop).

Most patients will be advised to avoid a suspect food completely for at least six months. After this many patients can get away with an occasional taste without symptoms, and some will succeed in re-introducing the food on a rotation diet, usually with at least a three-day cycle. Others may need to wait as much as two years before such experimentation is possible, and a few patients remain permanently sensitive, especially where milk products are involved.

SPECIALIZED TESTS IN CLINICAL ECOLOGY

Skin tests
- Patch tests (see p. 45)
- Intradermal injections of allergen – produce a weal which enlarges over the next few days if allergic, otherwise goes down. Accurate for pollens, dusts and spores, less so for food allergies. Time-consuming and expensive.

Blood tests
- RAST test (see p. 45)
- Cytotoxic test – involves exposing white blood cells to a series of suspected allergens and noting their reactions. Said to be more accurate than a RAST test but expensive and difficult to interpret.

Pulse tests
- Coca test – taking the pulse before and at intervals up to an hour after eating a suspect food. Any change (increase or decrease) of more than 10 beats per minute suggests allergy. Time-consuming but cheap.
- Auricular-cardiac reflex (ACR) – a sign derived from acupuncture involving movement of the strongest point of the wrist pulse on contact with the suspected food.

Electrical testing (Vega test)
Testing with specialized electrical equipment over certain acupuncture points, and noting fluctuations when suspect foods are placed onto a test plate on the control box. Rapid and cheap.

Another treatment which may be used is called 'Miller desensitization'. How it works is unexplained but it is reported to be effective. It stems from skin tests using injections of suspected allergens under the skin. Even people who do not react to a particular allergen often react to a dilution of it, a sort of 'homoeopathic symptom', for reasons unknown. If the solution is progressively diluted and increasing dilutions are injected at intervals over the next few hours, eventually a dilution

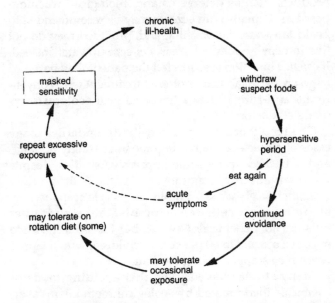

Fig. 4 Masked sensitivity
Adapted from 'Clinical Ecology' by Dr George T Lewith and Dr Julian N Kenyan, with permission

will be reached which produces no reaction in the skin.

This seems to obliterate the symptoms of the food sensitivity, and the patient may be able to eat small quantities of the food by first taking drops of that particular dilution under the tongue. After a couple of years it may be possible to stop using the drops without symptoms recurring. The technique is especially useful for people sensitive to common ingredients who would otherwise be confined to an extremely restricted diet. However it takes time and must be repeated for each allergy-provoking substance, and those with multiple sensitivities can find themselves needing many different drops, which eventually becomes impractical.

Clinical ecologists will also advise on avoiding common contact irritants, especially suspect domestic products such as detergents and 'biological' washing-powders. Patients with eczema may be recommended to avoid tap water for washing and, provided they do not live in heavily-polluted areas, collect rainwater instead. If *candida* infection is suspected the patient may be asked to go on a special diet, or offered treatment with conventional anti-fungal drugs (most clinical ecologists are qualified doctors).

The idea that allergy or sensitivity underlies many cases of atopic eczema has become increasingly popular, and is backed up by some impressive studies, despite the reservations of immune specialists. A drug called *sodium cromoglycate*, which blocks allergic responses by stopping mast-cells releasing histamine and other inflammatory chemicals (see p. 8, 54), has been shown to improve eczema in 60 per cent of children, who relapsed when they stopped taking the drug.

Many studies have shown that avoiding foods or chemicals incriminated by ecological methods in 'allergic' or auto-immune diseases helps a significant proportion of patients. Studies by conventional doctors have shown that about a quarter of children with eczema respond to dietary measures.

Biochemic tissue salts

These are supplements whose use is based on the philosophy that all diseases represent abnormalities of cell metabolism. That is, by the way that nutrients are taken up, utilized to carry out the functions of the cell and their waste-products excreted back into the system. If cell nutrition is adequate cell metabolism is normal. Conversely, if certain vital minerals are deficient metabolism is disturbed and disease may result. It can be corrected by taking supplements of the deficient mineral tissue salts.

The remedies are homoeopathically prepared (see p. 114), although they do not work on the like-cures-like principle but aim to correct imbalances and stimulate the immune system to promote healing. There are 12 individual remedies, based on various forms of the minerals calcium, potassium, iron, magnesium, sodium and silica, and a variety of combined preparations. The tablets are intended to dissolve under the tongue so entering the bloodstream directly without passing through the gut first:

- *Ferrum phosphate* for inflammation
- *Kali muriaticum* for skin scaling
- *Kali phosphate* for soreness, and for irritability and stress-related eczema
- *Kali sulphate* for dry skin or scaling and to maintain skin condition
- *Silica* helps skin-rashes
- Combination of *kali muriaticum, kali sulphate, calc sulphate* and *silica* aids skin ailments, dry skin and nappy rash.

Many natural therapists prescribe tissue salts, which are also available over-the-counter for self-help, and are recommended for a host of minor ailments such as colds, migraine, hay fever, stress-related illnesses and even sciatica. They are prepared homoeopathically so they are completely safe, even for babies and small children. The dose can be increased for more troublesome symptoms as there is no risk of overdose, although it should generally be halved for children. The only caution is that as the tablet base is made from lactose (milk sugar), those who are lactose intolerant should not take them. Some people swear by them even though there is very little research to support their effectiveness. Certainly they seem to be harmless.

Ayurvedic medicine

Ayurveda is an Indian philosophy based on belief in universal life energy (see p. 99), in India called *prana*, with good health relying on balance and harmony of various forces. Traditional ayurvedic medicine is preventive, aiming to correct imbalances before they lead to disease. Imbalances may result from an individual's constitution, from eating badly or improperly prepared food, from sleeping or sexual difficulties, strong emotions, lack of exercise or the effects of climate.

Many Indian-trained ayurvedic practitioners now practise in the west, and some doctors have taken additional training in ayurvedic techniques. They can be used to treat any ailment, but adherents claim especial success with stress-related illnesses and chronic conditions such as arthritis, asthma and eczema.

As in conventional medicine, diseases may be treated by both drugs and surgery, although most medicines are based on traditional herbal remedies. Treatment relies heavily on changes in diet and lifestyle, as well as specific nutritional remedies, and also incorporates *yoga*, breathing exercises, massage, meditation and various religious rituals.

Practitioners place great importance on both the content and preparation of food, believing that foods such as milk, fat and fibre can produce the same purifying effect as fasting (which may also be recommended), and help to reduce anxiety. In contrast, meat, spices and sweets are believed to increase energy levels, so help lethargy and depression. Food should be appropriate to the season and time of day, eaten slowly and chewed well while in a relaxed state of mind.

One controversial technique is encouraging people to drink their own urine. This reportedly clears eczema overnight in some cases, in theory because of the presence of the patient's own antibodies (western medicine would dispute this since antibodies are proteins which are not present in urine in healthy people).

Success is partly dependent on acceptance of the cultural and religious beliefs of ayurveda, and on the willingness to adopt specific lifestyle practices, which may be hard for those from different cultures.

Naturopathy

Naturopathy is based on the healing powers of nature, hence the old term 'Nature Cure'. It uses a complex mix of nutritional therapy, folk remedies, exercise and psychological techniques. Naturopathic training covers the same specialities as conventional medicine, and naturopaths often work side-by-side with conventional doctors, some having a dual qualification. Many also use some conventional techniques and other natural therapies (especially osteopathy) provided they fit the aim of helping the body to help itself. Most naturopaths work in private practice, and some run clinics in health farms or spas.

Naturopaths see illness as bodily imbalances so that while they recognize external causes of disease, such as infections, these are regarded as secondary to the internal, emotional or lifestyle factors which made the person vulnerable. As with homoeopathy, symptoms are seen as the body's attempts to cure itself, and there may be a healing crisis (see p. 115) as they resurface while the body recovers. Naturopathy emphasizes good nutrition and exercise, living naturally and thinking positively.

It is said to be effective for many chronic conditions, including both skin disorders and allergies, and can help if a sufferer also feels anxious or stressed.

Eczema is seen as a stress-related condition in which heredity and allergies may play a role, and many naturopaths take literally the Greek meaning of the word, 'to boil over'. They view the dry skin and expanded surface blood vessels of eczema as representing the body's attempts to get rid of heat, and therapy concentrates on 'keeping cool' both nutritionally and psychologically. Recommended treatment could include

- avoiding dietary stimulants like tea, coffee and spicy foods
- avoiding smoking and alcohol
- cutting down on processed foods, red meat, meat fats, sugar, saturated fats (butter, cream), cholesterol (eggs, cheese)
- eating raw fruit and vegetables as much as possible
- eating more pulses (like lentils), wholegrain bread and pasta and oily fish (mackerel, sardines)
- ensuring adequate rest and daily relaxation
- adopting some form of regular relaxation if under stress such as massage, yoga, meditation or self-hypnosis
- skin care with almond, avocado or wheatgerm oil
- encouraging a calm and contented home environment for children (such as excluding noisy or violent films or videos, avoiding persistent criticism and encouraging mild exercise without allowing them to get overexcited).

People often instinctively stop eating when they are seriously ill ('feed a cold and starve a fever'), and many naturopaths use fasting or liquid-only diets for short periods. Some advocate B vitamin supplements or high-dose vitamin C (1000mg – or one gram – or more a day).

If you wish to try fasting yourself (and many people swear by a regular fast one day a week to give the body a rest and a chance for a clear-out of toxins), remember it is vital to keep up a good intake of liquids (humans do not last long without water). The effects can be unpleasant, with headaches, bowel disturbances, bad breath, nausea or headaches, and nutritional imbalances can develop. Prolonged fasts (more than a couple of days), or fasts in children, should only ever be undertaken with the supervision of a qualified dietician or doctor.

The broad approach and general philosophy of naturopathy make it likely that at least part of the overall treatment will produce some improvement for a condition like eczema, and unlikely that any serious side-effects will result. It does, however, require a similar open-mindedness on the part of the patient, and a willingness to adapt one's lifestyle accordingly.

CHAPTER 9

Therapies for healing the skin

Other whole-system approaches

If you're taking care of your skin, you've avoided any known contacts, dealt with stress and changed your diet yet you still get flare-ups of eczema don't despair. There are still several natural healing systems or therapies left to try which have helped many people to reduce the severity of their eczema and lessen the frequency of attacks, irrespective of what triggers the symptoms. The most convincing are:

- Acupuncture
- Acupressure
- Reflexology
- Western herbal medicine
- Chinese herbal medicine
- Homoeopathy.

All except western herbal medicine depend for their effect on a belief in the invisible 'healing energy' and all except western herbal medicine and homoeopathy are based on Oriental ideas of healing systems. The choice of therapy now depends on how effective it might be in your case, and how well it fits with your personal preferences and beliefs.

Acupuncture

This is a form of traditional Chinese medicine which has been written about for more than 2000 years. It is based on the Oriental belief in an energy or life force present both within the human body and throughout the universe called *qi* or *chi* in China, *ki* in Japan, and *prana* in India. The flow and balance of energy is considered crucial to health and vitality. Disturbances or blockages lead to disharmony and disease and can result from inherited susceptibilities, climate, dietary excesses, strong emotions, drugs, infections, and over- or under-indulgence in exercise, work and sex.

The use of needles inserted along the 12 channels (or 'meridians') where *qi* flows through the body is believed to restore balance and flow of energy. The various meridians are said to influence different bodily organs and systems (not necessarily the ones they are named after).

As well as needling, practitioners may use moxibustion, in which a burning herb (*mugwort*) is placed at the head of the needle, or held on a stick near the acupuncture point. More recently, techniques of electro-acupuncture have been developed in which a weak electric current is passed down the needles, or applied direct to the skin surface without the use of needles at all. Several devices are now on sale for people to perform electro-acupuncture at home.

Numerous studies have shown acupuncture to be effective for relieving pain and nausea, and it is now used in many western hospitals for this purpose. The research has shown that it stimulates the body to release chemicals called *endorphins*. These have a morphine-like action and are released automatically in response to injury or pain as a form of natural pain-killer. Endorphins also promote feelings of well-being, stimulate healing, and may help defend against allergic reactions.

Chinese research has also demonstrated success with various chronic ailments including arthritis, high blood pressure, depression, anxiety, gut disorders, asthma, eczema, hay fever, infertility, headaches and menstrual problems. There are no known side-effects provided sterile needles are used (as by law in most countries they must be) to guard against infection. The needles are made usually of steel so should not provoke allergic reactions, but occasionally of gold.

Practitioners see eczema as linked with exposure to heat, cold, wind and damp, and as a failure of bodily elimination processes (both physical and emotional), resulting in built-up toxins or suppressed emotions expressed through the skin.

There has been little research in the West to assess acupuncture in eczema, but one fascinating study has shown that some skin-rashes occur along the lines of the meridians, which offers support for their existence and influence on skin disease. There is also a phenomenon in which, during needling, a few people experience sensations along the line of the meridian (even though they may not know where or even what it is), and those who do seem to gain more benefit.

Practitioners say that more than 80 per cent of patients with skin diseases are either cured or substantially (more than 50 per cent) improved, and traditional practitioners in China claim even higher rates of up to 99 per cent.

There are acupuncture points all over the body but the arms, legs, hands and feet are most often used so you do not necessarily need to undress for needles to be inserted. The point of insertion may be at some distance from the skin rash. The needles are extremely thin and after a slight prick as they are inserted most people feel either nothing at all or a slight tingling sensation. The needles are usually left in place for 20 minutes or more, when you should feel no more than heaviness of the limbs and a sense of relaxation.

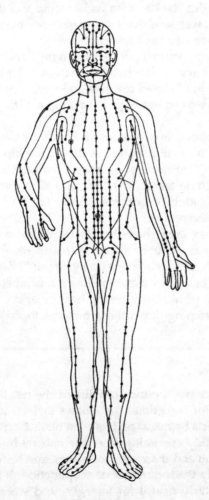

Fig. 5 Acupuncture meridians

Judith's story

Judith, 46, went to an acupuncturist with a hip problem. A former horserider, she feared she might have arthritis. But she had also had eczema and dry skin for years, was sensitive to dust, and her mother and teenage son also have skin problems.

"The acupuncturist put needles in my hands, ankles and the back of my head", she says. "It sounds revolting but I closed my eyes and never felt a thing. In fact, it was so relaxing that a couple of times I fell asleep."

It took about three months of weekly treatment sessions, with moxibustion as well, for the hip pain to go away. "But almost at once I realized my skin wasn't itching any more either, and after three treatments a patch of eczema on my leg had disappeared," she reports.

Two years later she is hardly troubled by eczema but has had a couple of repeat treatments for occasional recurrences brought on by stress: "I hated taking pills, and acupuncture seems a much better way to get my whole body feeling healthy again, instead of just damping down the symptoms to make them bearable."

Acupressure

Acupressure is acupuncture without the needles, using the hands (or sometimes the elbows or feet) to achieve similar effects by massage. It is even older than acupuncture, probably stemming from the natural human tendency to rub and massage sore places, and some believe it is actually the forerunner of acupuncture. It is said to be particularly useful for allergies and stress-related problems.

There are several sub-varieties or schools of acupressure:

Do-In
This combines acupressure with exercise and breathing routines.

Jin Shen (or sometimes *Jin Shin*)
This uses more prolonged massage (several minutes) of a series of selected acupuncture points. There are several forms which often tag a third word onto the name such as *Jin Shen Do*.

Shen Tao
This uses acupressure as part of a natural or 'holistic' approach within traditional Chinese medicine.

Shiatsu
Developed in Japan where it is often used for preventive healthcare, this is the most popular variant. The word means 'finger pressure' and the technique uses short bursts of pressure (a few seconds each) along the meridians. The acupuncture points are called *tsubos*, and treatment is believed to affect circulation, lymphatic flow, hormonal balance and the nervous system as well as body energy flow.

In theory acupressure offers very similar benefits to acupuncture although little research has been done to prove this. It is certainly very helpful for relieving symptoms of stress and practitioners claim good results with eczema, although results may take longer to achieve than with acupuncture.

Most therapists give a general massage to find and work on any sensitive areas before moving on to specific treatment points, so it is usually carried out lying down. You should wear loose clothing but usually do not need to undress. A session can be as short as 15 minutes but usually takes about an hour. Many people find the massage deeply relaxing and some even fall asleep, while others emerge energized and refreshed.

Reflexology

Reflexology is a system of foot massage which is claimed to have been widely practised in most ancient cultures from China to North America. Like acupressure, with which it has much in common, it may be even older than acupuncture (perhaps 5000 years). Traditional Chinese medicine is linked with *Taoism*, a philosophy which views all things as reflecting and containing some part of a larger whole. Hence the function of the body can be seen in a specific part, such as the face or feet. In reflexology the feet are seen as mirrors of the body, with different areas corresponding to the various body systems.

Like acupuncture, it sees disease as stemming from blockage of energy channels (six of the main acupuncture meridians run through the feet). Foot massage is used to restore energy flow and stimulate blood and lymph flow to replenish and de-toxify the body. For eczema massage might be given to the areas related to the digestive system, liver, kidneys, thyroid, adrenal and pituitary glands as well as the parts of skin affected.

Practitioners claim reflexology can be used for similar chronic ailments to acupuncture, and for more serious conditions such as heart disease or multiple sclerosis. It is extremely relaxing which may well help in stress-related conditions. There are usually no side-effects, but sometimes improvement is accompanied by symptoms of clearing (see 'healing crisis', p. 115). For example, treating a respiratory problem can cause a temporary flow of mucus.

There are three main variations in use:

Reflex Zone Therapy (or sometimes simply 'Zone therapy') This is a derivative devised in the early years of the twentieth century which sees energy as flowing through ten areas or zones of the body to points in the hands and feet. It was first used as a pain-killing technique. It is not

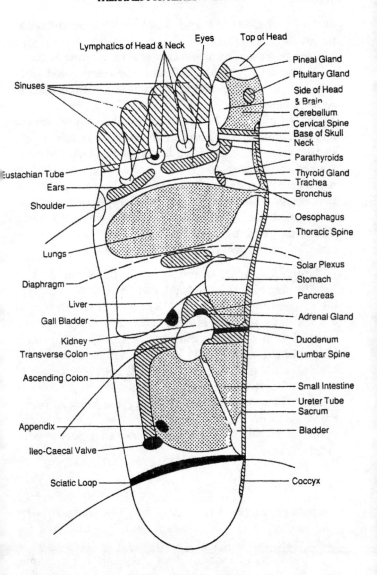

Fig. 6 Reflexology zones on the right foot

suitable for everyone and should not be used during pregnancy.

The Metamorphic Technique This sees foot points as corresponding with prenatal influences, where stored traumas can create emotional difficulties which lead to illness in later life.

Vacuflex Reflexology is a high-tech version in which the feet are stimulated by vacuum pressure rather than touch. It uses a special pair of felt boots from which the air is sucked out to treat the whole foot at once in only five minutes. When the boots are removed markings left on the feet for a few minutes tell the therapist which points on the meridians need further treatment with special suction pads (reminiscent of 'cupping' in traditional medicine). Its practitioners claim it helps eczema and allergies.

Although the theory of reflexology is based on more or less the same ideas as acupuncture there is no comparable evidence to back it up. There have been no formal clinical trials yet of its efficacy in disease states and conventional medicine remains extremely sceptical. However the technique is harmless and is undoubtedly both pleasant and deeply relaxing. It has been shown to reduce anxiety and stress to a greater extent than counselling and so may be useful for eczema brought on by emotions. If no improvement occurs after a few sessions you may do better by changing therapies or seeing your family doctor.

Herbal medicine

Herbalism is generally regarded as the oldest healing skill known. It is still the main source of medicine for more than four-fifths of the world's population and is the forerunner of modern drug medicine. For example, the heart drug *digitalis* comes from foxgloves, the active ingredient of *aspirin* is found in willow-bark, *quinine* (used to treat malaria) comes from the bark of the *cinchona* tree and opium poppies yield *morphine*. Researchers are still exploring the potential for cancers and other serious diseases of newly-discovered herbal remedies from the Amazon rain-forests.

Gradually the drugs industry has moved from extracting specific chemicals from plants to mass-producing synthetic substitutes to generating novel drugs entirely in the laboratory. Today most drugs are composed of a single synthetic chemical, although about one in seven are still plant-based.

By contrast, a herbal medicine (which may not be a herb in the kitchen sense but any plant part found to be effective) may contain thousands of ingredients from the natural plant. The effects are much more complex and often seem remarkably well-tuned to human needs, even if less well-understood. For instance, a herbal remedy may relieve several symptoms which often occur together, or potential side-effects from the active ingredient may be balanced by others which counteract them. Herbal remedies derived from plants growing in particular parts of the world are often effective against diseases common to that region (but not so effective against similar ailments elsewhere).

Herbal remedies can be chewed, swallowed, applied to the skin, inhaled, put in bathwater or in douches and suppositories. They may be taken directly, cooked with, given as infusions or herbal teas, made into tablets, creams, ointments, poultices or liquid extracts. You can grow your own, buy them as plants or pre-prepared remedies, or visit a trained herbalist. Modern herbalists usually prescribe herbs in concentrated liquid form (tinctures or decoctions) which can be taken by the spoonful, but some use elixirs, cordials, teas, pills, ointments, bath additives or poultices, and a few may advise taking fresh or dried herbs neat.

Remember that while plant remedies are generally gentle, effective and safe some are poisonous. So herbal medicines should always be treated with respect. If you want to treat yourself, check out the safety, dose and method of preparation in a good herbal book first (see appendix B), and never use herbs in pregnancy without professional advice.

Herbalists view eczema as related to allergies (especially to dairy products), nutritional factors, stress and emotional tension or problems with elimination, such as chronic constipation. Advice on diet will usually be given, often with suggestions about exercise or combating stress and emotional problems as well. Practitioners view symptoms as the body's way of trying to restore its own internal balance, so the function of herbal remedies is to aid self-healing and promote overall health. Prescriptions are individual, so yours may not match that of someone else with eczema, and may also vary on different occasions. Usually for a condition like eczema several consultations will be needed. The first usually takes about an hour, while return visits can be much shorter.

There is no doubt that some herbal medicines can be as effective and quick-acting as the modern drugs derived from them. Others by their nature are more gentle remedies which take time to work. Many traditional herbal remedies are used within conventional medicine. For example, *peppermint* is an ingredient of many medicines for upset stomachs. *Feverfew*, a herbal remedy used for centuries for headaches and arthritis, has been found effective in migraine. *Garlic* has been shown to have anti-infective properties and to reduce high blood pressure.

While there has been no formal measurement of the success of herbal treatments overall in eczema there is no doubt that many sufferers do benefit, and one traditional remedy in particular has been found to be so successful that it has been adopted by conventional medicine.

Herbal remedies useful against ezcema

There are many mild herbal remedies said to help skin complaints or eczema, and other remedies which may be useful for associated symptoms such as stress, sleeplessness or respiratory complaints. For example:

- *Calendula* or *marigold* tea or ointment relieves itching, blistering and flaking and may help prevent eczema attacks. It is also good for the complexion.
- A poultice made of fresh green *cabbage* leaves (especially Savoy cabbage), warmed and crushed then layered on the skin under a bandage overnight relieves eczema
- *Chickweed* infusion, oil or ointment can help itching
- *Blackberry, raspberry, loganberry* or *elder-leaf* teas strengthen the skin, and may be used externally to help eczema
- *Goldenseal* relieves eczema symptoms and speeds healing: mix the powder with honey to eat, or with warm water to paint on the skin
- *St John's Wort* oil rubbed into the skin relieves inflammation and blistering (and also deters insects)
- *Walnut* leaf tea has been used for eczema and externally for skin eruptions
- *Nettle* tea helps skin complaints associated with poor elimination
- *Almond* oil is good for dry skin and so soothes itching
- *Camomile* tea is calming and soothing and makes an excellent bedtime drink to promote rest and sleep
- *Parsley, dandelion-root* and *red clover* help maintain vigour and combat stress.

Evening primrose oil

One of the best known herbal remedies today, evening primrose oil (EPO) is now available on prescription as well as from chemists and healthfood shops for the treatment of premenstrual syndrome and eczema (see chapter 5). EPO, borage (starflower) and blackcurrant seed oil contain *gamma linoleic* acid (GLA), one of the essential fatty acids, a group of oils which play a vital role in all body cells. GLA (and, perhaps, other fatty acids) seems to be deficient in people with atopic eczema so replacing stores by taking EPO could help the underlying cause of the disease.

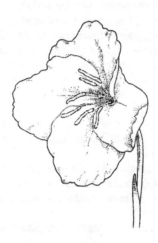

Fig. 7 The Evening primrose flower

EPO is particularly useful in childhood eczema. It is available as a liquid, although over-the-counter preparations are not intended for children under seven. For small children you should see your doctor who may prescribe a special version. EPO may also help adults and strengthen the skin in contact eczema. One study even showed it helped cats with skin disease. However you may need to use it for up to three months before you see any results, and you need to take quite a lot (up to six capsules daily) which can be expensive.

There seem to be no serious side-effects but a few users report nausea, indigestion or headache. It should not be used in anyone with epilepsy except under medical supervision.

Chinese herbal medicine

Chinese herbal medicine, like acupuncture, is part of traditional Chinese medicine, and so is based on the philosophy of body energy balance. Unlike western herbalists, with a relatively limited plant 'menu' (a few hundred) and usually using remedies based on single plants or a small combination, oriental medicine draws on a range of more than 4,000 herbs made up in various complex formulas.

An individual mixture is usually prescribed as dried herbs to be freshly brewed and drunk, as a tea, daily for several weeks or months, depending on the severity of the condition. For skin conditions practitioners may also use herbal mixes externally, in creams and lotions or as a solution for washing or using in the bath, for short-term symptom relief while the herbs begin to work internally.

With the backing of western medicine, research in China to support its effectiveness and other research projects underway in the UK, Chinese herbal medicine appears one of the most promising remedies for eczema, even for severe cases not helped by the most powerful conventional treatments. Its use in the West is perhaps the most exciting development in the treatment of eczema for decades.

Homoeopathy

Homoeopathy is a complete system of medicine developed in the late eighteenth century, but based on principles suggested by Hippocrates in the fifth century BC. It holds that symptoms are the body's attempts to fight

The '10-herb' Chinese herbal cure found in Soho

Chinese herbal medicine as a treatment for eczema received an exciting boost in 1993 when British skin specialists decided to investigate remarkable improvements reported by patients who visited a traditional Chinese practitioner working in London's Soho district. Having watched her work, they realized that although she used many different herbs in different combinations, certain ingredients featured time and again. Together they developed a fixed formula called 'Zemaphyte' containing ten herbs at a relatively constant dose (no mean feat in dealing with tea-leaves), and put it to the test in two formal trials at top London hospitals.

In both adults and children with severe atopic eczema which had failed to respond to conventional treatments four weeks therapy with the herbal mixture, brewed fresh daily from pre-prepared sachets, produced significant reductions in average scores of redness and surface skin damage, with less itching and better sleep in most patients, and no serious side-effects. There are now plans to try to make the formulation into a pill to make it more convenient to take and avoid the nasty taste of the teas.

While the ten-herb treatment is not yet generally available traditional Chinese herbalists, who often use many of the same ingredients, claim success rates of 80 per cent or more (by which they mean that 80 per cent of the affected skin is cleared) in most patients, with complete cure in some. Most patients are advised to give the herbs at least three months trial, and a full course may last up to four to six months, during which the patient needs to return every week or so for further assessment and repeat prescriptions.

Some centres offer a few standard herb combinations as pills to be used for maintenance treatment, or if someone is going away or for some other reason cannot brew the tea fresh daily – but since these are not 'individualized' to the patient they may not work as well or as rapidly.

Julie's story

Julie is six and has had extensive eczema since she was three months old. While she was a baby attacks cleared up fairly readily with steroid creams from her family doctor, so although it was quite noticeable on her cheeks her mother felt it was 'liveable with'. Then her second child was born, when Julie was nearly three. "She seemed to cope with the new baby in other ways but the eczema went bezerk, virtually every inch of her body was covered".

It got to the stage where Julie's parents were taking it in turns to stay in her room overnight, holding her hands to stop her 'ripping herself to pieces' scratching. Stronger and stronger steroids were all her doctor could offer. Cutting out dairy foods did not help, nor did homoeopathy. Then her father saw a newspaper article about London's Chi Centre which specializes in Chinese herbal treatments for skin diseases.

"The tea she had to take was the most disgusting-smelling, vile-tasting brown liquid, and took ages to brew up. We had real trouble getting her to take it, even mixing it with her favourite drinks. Then the centre put us in touch with another family, and Julie spoke to the other child on the `phone who said yes, the tea tasted really yuckky but it had made her skin better. We kept going and within a few days she was sleeping at nights. Gradually her skin improved. She took the tea for 18 months altogether. We finished two years ago. Since then she's had the odd small patch of eczema which goes away rapidly by using evening primrose oil cream, and she hasn't needed steroids for three years. The treatment wasn't cheap but it was well worth it – at that stage we would have done anything."

disease, so instead of suppressing them treatment should work with them to assist the body's own healing resources.

Homoeopathic remedies consist of minutely small doses of substances which, if given at full strength to a healthy person, would cause similar symptoms to those of the patient. This is the 'Principle of Similars', or like-cures-like. Conventional or allopathic medicine, by contrast, aims to counteract the symptoms – a cure of opposites (the words 'homoeopathy' and 'allopathy' come from the Greek *homoios* meaning 'similar', *allos* meaning 'different' and *pathos* meaning 'suffering').

Remedies are derived from plants, minerals and metals prepared by steeping in alcohol to create a 'mother tincture', then progressively diluting this, shaking vigorously each time (known as 'succussion'). In some cases toxins or antigens like pollens, animal furs or house dust mite are used to produce specific homoeopathic 'antidotes' called *nosodes*.

The final solution is made into pills by adding sugar, and tablets are graded according to successive decimal (10-fold) or centesimal (100-fold) dilutions (usually written as, say, 'X6' or C6'). Homoeopaths hold that the more dilute the mixture the greater its potency. They believe that the process of dilution itself enhances the power of the remedy (called 'potentization'), and that the water retains a 'memory' or 'blueprint' of the original substance caused by the shaking.

Homoeopathy can be used to treat any condition, although practitioners stress that it is not a substitute for emergency treatment or urgent surgery. Practitioners often give a single dose of a homoeopathic remedy, then monitor the patient for a while, since any changes are said to show that the medicine has had an effect. However with chronic conditions like eczema further doses may be given if nothing happens, or alternative remedies prescribed as the overall picture changes.

Homoeopaths believe that the most long-standing symptoms are the last to go and that cure occurs from inside out. So, for example, disease of internal organs may be displaced to the skin in the course of healing. Patients are warned that they may get worse before they get better (a 'healing crisis'), with old symptoms reappearing before they are finally resolved, and that if this proves too severe further advice should be sought at once.

Homoeopathic remedies are prescribed according to a complex assessment of someone's personality, mood, reactions and habits as well as their symptoms. Eczema is seen as an outward sign of an underlying disorder, so although over-the-counter remedies are available professional help is really advisable.

Also, while generally homoeopathic and conventional treatment can be carried out side-by-side, homoeopaths believe steroid creams reduce the body's own healing powers and so may make homoeopathy less effective. Many practitioner organizations therefore recommend that people with eczema see a medically-trained homoeopath so that steroid use can be dealt with as well.

Because some practitioners use homoeopathic preparations to 'immunize' against certain diseases, homoeopaths themselves have become involved in the sometimes heated controversy about childhood immunizations which is often a source of anxiety to parents of atopic children. Some natural therapists believe that the conventional view (see p. 38) does not take full account of the potential long-term hazards of certain immunizations. While many endorse conventional immunizations against diseases like tetanus and polio some feel that the balance of benefits versus risks for others, especially whooping cough and mumps-measles-rubella (MMR) vaccines, is less clear-cut. Some practitioners may there-

fore recommend homoeopathic immunization instead.
Such decisions cause many parents great anguish. The
debate is too complex to cover in detail here but a med-
ically- qualified homoeopath will appreciate both sides
of the argument and will generally be happy to discuss it
with you at length.

Common homoeopathic remedies for eczema

Although two people with the same condition will not necessarily receive the same treatment some common remedies
used for eczema are:

- For cracked and oozing skin which burns and itches:
  Graphites. If the itch is worse at night: *Petroleum*
- For weeping crusted eczema made worse by damp:
  Dulcamara
- For dry itchy skin made worse by cold: *Arsenicum album*
- For intense itching made worse by heat: *Sulphur*
- For eczema with greasy skin and raw patches, especially
  around hairlines: *Natrum muriaticum*
- For eczema symptoms associated with constipation:
  Calcarea carbonicum.

Homoeopathy occupies a curious position in medicine in
that its philosophy is almost completely opposed to conventional medicine yet it is practised by doctors. In Britain
it is the only form of natural therapy to have been readily
available on the free state National Health Service since its
inception in 1948, and more than 2000 UK doctors are
trained in homoeopathy. The British Royal Family's well-
known support and long-time use of homoeopathy have
also helped to maintain its status and increase its popularity. But many doctors remain extremely suspicious.

A particularly common objection is that the most
potent homoeopathic remedies are so dilute that they
may contain no molecules of the original substance at
all. There is no scientifically acceptable theory of how
they might work (although recent attempts have been

made to explain 'memory' for the substances in terms of the physics of water molecule structure), and formal studies of homoeopathy have given mixed results and are not always repeatable.

While conceding that homoeopathic remedies are therefore extremely safe, even for babies and small children, many doctors dismiss any improvements seen as 'placebo effects' (mind over matter). However, many vets use homoeopathy and studies have shown benefits such as preventing stillbirth in pigs, and even responses in plants, which can hardly be placebo effects. Other successful experiments include:

- Numerous studies in laboratory tissue, animals and humans showing changes in biological measurements such as hormone levels, enzymes and immune response
- Evidence of anti-viral and analgesic (pain-killing) activity
- A controversial study published in the prestigious science journal *Nature* showing laboratory evidence of distinct changes in certain body cells triggered by a homoeopathic preparation, with results reproduced in several centres
- Many studies showing benefit in chronic conditions like arthritis, hay fever, fibrositis and migraine, and even acute diseases like influenza.

One study showed that three-quarters of adults and nearly 90 per cent of children with atopic eczema were significantly improved after homoeopathic treatment (homoeopaths say children are easier to treat because the disease is less long-standing). However the adults were treated for an average of nearly two years, the children for two and a half years, during which time spontaneous improvement could have occurred in many. There was no comparison with other treatments or with no treatment at all to suggest how much of the improvement was directly due to homoeopathy.

Another study did compare homoeopathy with conventional treatment in children with atopic eczema and found no difference. This implies that homoeopathy can be as effective as steroids without their potential dangers.

Michael's story

Michael was a very unhappy 10-year-old with dry, scabby eczema covering his whole body. This had started after his uncle, his only 'father figure', died. When his mother first brought him he slunk in, looking downcast, and sat shuffling his feet, answering questions briefly and dully. Finally, he admitted he was being teased at school and dreaded taking part in gym classes because of his skin, something he had not told his mother before.

She did not want any more steroid creams (which hadn't helped in the past anyway) but was desperate for some treatment to lessen his misery and the intense itching which was keeping him awake at night. The homoeopath prescribed a remedy to take account of the boy's grief about his uncle. For a week his eczema got worse and his mother was on the 'phone daily but she was persuaded to wait and see.

Gradually the skin improved, and although the homoeopath saw him every month nothing more was prescribed (homoeopaths say that once some change occurs the healing has begun so no further remedies are needed – something patients often do not expect). After five months the eczema was nearly clear and Michael was a changed boy: lively, talkative and making eye contact when he spoke excitedly of enjoying his new swimming classes.

CHAPTER 10

How to find and choose a natural therapist

Tips and guidelines for seeking out reliable help

Although all forms of natural medicine are enjoying an upsurge in popularity in most Western countries it is not always as easy as it might be to find the right therapist to help. Once you've decided which therapy is right for you there is no unified system comparable with conventional medicine to point you in the right direction. This means you have to take much more responsibility for tracking down a suitable therapist and checking that whoever you intend to visit is qualified, experienced and, preferably, good at making people better.

A personal recommendation from someone you know is almost always the best way of finding the right person. If you don't know anyone who has reported positive results with natural therapists ask around among friends, neighbours and colleagues. A recommendation from someone with the same problem can be especially encouraging, and if you belong to a patient support group you will almost certainly find some people within it who have tried natural techniques. In Britain, for instance, the National Eczema Society has local groups in many areas where you can meet other sufferers and trawl for information.

If you still draw a blank, try your local doctor's clinic (or even your dentist for major therapies like acupuncture and homoeopathy). Not all will give a helpful reception to this kind of request, but many are surprisingly broadminded – and you will almost certainly not be the first patient to ask.

Most clinics will at least be aware of natural therapists practising in the area (often because patients have told them about successful treatment), and may be prepared to give you the names of the most popular, even if they will not formally recommend one. Some practices nowadays have at least one doctor who is trained in some form of natural technique, or have visiting natural therapists working in their clinics which may allow you to get free treatment in countries with a state health service. Many other practices are sympathetic to the principle of natural medicine and willing to refer patients to other local therapists.

If that doesn't work try other local sources such as libraries and healthfood shops: the names of successful local therapists are usually well-known. Therapists usually know of each other too, so if you get a recommendation which is not for the therapy of your choosing, try asking that therapist for the names of other therapists who practise nearby.

Alternatively, many larger towns have a natural health centre which may have several therapists with different skills working there. The very best enable you to have an initial consultation in which your case can be considered by a panel of therapists to select the best forms of treatment, although this multi-disciplinary approach is still relatively new and so hard to find. Again, if the therapy you want is not on offer, the centre may know other therapists working locally.

Centres and individual therapists may be listed in local *Yellow Pages*, newspapers, libraries, citizens advice and information centres. Or you can contact national organizations for natural medicine, or national therapist bodies, who can usually supply (sometimes for a fee) a list of local members, as well as more general information. Such organizations are listed in the resources section at the end of this book (Appendix A).

---

10 ways of finding a therapist

- Word of mouth (usually by far the best recommendation)
- Doctor's surgery or clinic
- Local patient support groups: for example, UK National Eczema Society (see Appendix A)
- Local natural health centres
- Health farms and beauty treatment centres
- Healthfood shop noticeboards or ask staff
- National organizations of therapists (see Appendix A)
- Computer networks (you need a modem)
- Local *Yellow Pages*, newspapers or magazines
- Public libraries and information centres.

Selecting a therapist

You may be lucky enough to find direct guidance in finding a therapist you feel comfortable with, and of whose background you are sure. If you have had to do more research and have less in the way of personal recommendation, you will probably have armed yourself with a list of possibilities but may be unsure how to proceed from there.

In selecting a therapist bear in mind that while most natural therapists are well-trained, caring and competent people there is no particular disincentive to crooks and charlatans setting themselves up with little training, especially in Britain which is almost alone in the world in having almost no restrictions on who may practice what when it comes to natural therapies. It is because of this that the British Medical Association in its 1993 report on natural medicine recommended that anyone seeking the help of a non-conventional therapist asks some searching questions of the therapist, including:

- the therapist's qualifications and training
- how long they have been in practice
- whether they belong to a recognized professional body with a laid down code of conduct, and
- whether they have professional indemnity insurance.

Always feel free to ask such questions before booking an appointment, and steer clear of anyone who sounds vague or shifty about answering. You want to be wary of being treated by someone who has done only one weekend course in the therapy they are offering.

Checking professional organizations

If a therapist belongs to a professional organization, a good starting point is to get more information about the organization itself. Questions which are useful to ask include:

- When was it founded?
- How many members does it have?
- Does it have members nationwide? Groups which have been going for 50 years and have many members are likely to be better organized and well-accepted than those started last week in someone's living room.
- Is it part of a larger network of professional organizations? Bodies representing the major therapies often belong to an umbrella organization supporting the aims and standards of natural medicine in general. Groups which 'do their own thing' entirely may be less likely to adhere to recognized professional and ethical standards.
- Does it accept only members with recognized qualifications? If so, what are they? Large professional bodies

may be linked with colleges which train therapists, or set standards to oversee training. However, beware small organizations closely allied with one particular school or college: they may not have independent assessment of qualifications.

- Does it have a code of conduct, a complaints mechanism and disciplinary procedures for members who fail to conform to laid down standards?
- Is it a charity, educational trust or private company? Charities and trusts should exist to promote the therapy and serve the interests of members of the public. Private companies may be more interested in financial rewards.
- Are members covered by professional indemnity insurance against accident or malpractice? This is an important safeguard for you, and implies an overall professionalism and concern for patient welfare.

Checking training and qualifications

Next, you may want more details about the therapist's qualifications. Ideally, information from a therapist organization would describe recognized qualifications and explain what the letters after a therapist's name mean. If not, you need to ask the organization for an explanation, including:

- How long is the training?
- Is it full or part-time?
- Does it include seeing patients under supervision? Qualifications which are purely theoretical do not tell you much about someone's ability to treat people, and make it less likely that the therapist has had a substantial training.
- Is the qualification recognized? If so, by whom?

If you are interested in one of the major therapies, finding a medically-qualified therapist is an added safeguard if you are unsure or nervous about natural treatment. There are many doctors trained in homoeopathy, herbalism or acupuncture (but not many in flower remedies or aromatherapy), and if you live near a large city you should have no trouble finding a doctor with one of these specialised interests. Elsewhere you may have to travel further afield. Again, organizations which can help are listed in Appendix A.

Making the choice

A final selection, once you have assured yourself of each therapist's background, may depend on intuition and on trying them out. The scale and degree of luxuriousness of a practice may suggest that someone is popular or financially successful, but don't necessarily tell you whether they are any good. However if the surroundings 'feel wrong', or the therapist or practice staff make you feel uncomfortable, be guided by your feelings. Never be afraid to walk out or cancel appointments if you are not happy with the person, the place or the treatment.

Cautions

- If you are female, feel free to check whether you will be chaperoned if you need to undress, and to ask for someone of the same sex to be present if this makes you feel more comfortable. If the therapist says no, leave. It should go without saying that any sexual advances made by a therapist are unethical. This should never happen, but if anything makes you uneasy on that score, leave at once.
- You should never, ever stop drug treatment suddenly

without first discussing it with your doctor, and be extremely wary of any therapist who advises you to do so.

- Most natural therapists practise privately, and you should expect to pay the going rate for a professional consultation (although many therapists offer concessions to children or those on low incomes). But beware of anyone who asks for sums of money 'up front', and also of anyone who 'promises' you a 'cure'.

What to do if things go wrong

The most common reason for people to feel dissatisfied is if the treatment has not made them better. If so, first ask yourself whether you have given it a fair trial. Did you go into it with a positive outlook? Have you followed all the recommendations? Have you kept going for long enough? Many natural therapies take time to work, and some may even make you feel worse before you get better.

Next, do you feel the therapist was genuinely trying to help? No therapy can guarantee to be one hundred per cent successful, and you may be one of the unlucky ones who needs to look elsewhere for help.

However, if for any reason (whether the treatment was successful or not) you feel the therapist is incompetent, caused you harm, took risks or acted unprofessionally or unethically you should do something, if only to protect future patients. The sort of actions you can take are:

- Discuss it with the therapist if you feel you can – he or she may be unaware of the problem and only too ready to put it right once it is pointed out.
- Tell whoever recommended you, and anyone else you know you think could be affected. Ultimately this is

the most effective sanction since bad therapists rapidly get a reputation and lose patients. (But beware of spreading false or malicious rumours or you could be at risk of legal action for defamation.)

- Report the therapist to his or her professional body. This is where knowing your therapist is a member of a body with laid down codes of conduct is invaluable. Unfortunately, in Britain at least, such bodies have little regulatory authority, and cannot stop someone practising even though they may expel them.

- If you are very unhappy and have a case against them you could sue the therapist. This is likely to prove expensive unless some criminal action is involved, in which case go to the police. Otherwise consult a lawyer or ask citizen's rights or advice bureaux for help.

Conclusion

Despite scare stories about the occasional unscrupulous or untrained therapist preying on gullible or desperate people most natural therapists are reputable professionals. They have put much time and money into their training and invest much care and attention in their practice. You do need to choose carefully, but that is no bad thing. Taking some responsibility for caring for your own health, and playing an active role in treatment, have been shown to aid healing. It's your body and your mind, and it makes sense to treat them well, and to spend time and effort selecting someone to help you care for them – whether that person is a conventional doctor or a natural therapist, or both.

Ultimately it is also up to you to assess the treatment in progress and decide whether it is helping you or not. If not move on – but do not give up hope. A different approach may work wonders.

You may have to shop around to find a therapy and a therapist to suit you, but anyone with eczema has a very good chance of finding some form of treatment which offers significant relief. It may also have other benefits in making you feel generally healthier, calmer, fitter – and in getting to know someone you trust who you and your family can turn to with health problems in future.

Glossary

Acute (of illness) Short-term.

Allergen A substance capable of inducing an allergic reaction.

Allergenic Allergy-provoking.

Allergy Symptoms due to an idiosyncratic immune reaction to a substance not normally identified as hostile by most people.

Asthma Allergic respiratory disease characterized by wheezy breathing due to narrowing of the air passages

Atopy/Atopic Allergic tendency which runs in families and gives increased risk of asthma, eczema and hay fever.

Candida Type of fungal (yeast) infection commonly known as thrush

Cell The basic 'building block' of all body tissues.

Chronic (of illness) Long-lasting.

Dermatitis Inflammation of the skin (used interchangeably with eczema).

Dermis The second, underlying layer of the skin.

Epidermis Outer of the two layers of skin.

hay fever An allergic reaction involving runny nose and sore eyes, commonly due to pollen exposure.

Histamine A chemical produced in the body and involved in allergic reactions.

Holistic Taking account of the whole person.

Melanin Skin pigment which protects against the sun's rays.

Placebo An inert substance, such as a chalk pill, which someone believes to contain an active drug. Often used to compare with the effect of drugs and medicines. May still yield benefits and side-effects, held to be of psychological origin, known as the 'placebo effect'.

Qi (or *chi*) In Oriental philosophy, the life energy circulating throughout the universe and flowing through the body (also known as *ki* in Japan, *prana* in India).

Sebaceous gland Gland in the skin producing sebum (grease).

Sebum The greasy secretion of the skin, produced in sebaceous glands.

Steroid A type of hormone. Some are produced naturally in the body, others are man-made and given as drugs.

Urticaria An allergic skin eruption, also known as nettle-rash or hives.

APPENDIX A

Useful organizations

The following listing of organizations is for information only and does not imply any endorsement, nor do the organizations listed necessarily agree with the views expressed in this book.

INTERNATIONAL

International Federation of Practitioners of Natural Therapeutics
46 Pulens Crescent
Sheet
Petersfield
Hampshire GU31 4DH, UK.
Tel 0730 266790
Fax 0730 260058

AUSTRALASIA

Australian Natural Therapists Association
PO Box 308
Melrose Park
South Australia 5039.
Tel 8297 9533
Fax 8297 0003

Australian Traditional Medicine Society
PO Box 442 *or*
Suite 3, First Floor,
120 Blaxland Road
Ryde
New South Wales 2112.
Australia.
Tel 2808 2825
Fax 2809 7570

New Zealand Natural Health Practitioners Accreditation Board
PO Box 37-491
Auckland, New Zealand.
Tel 9625 9966

NORTH AMERICA

American Association of Naturopathic Physicians
2800 East Madison Street, Suite 200
Seattle
Washington 98112, USA
or
PO Box 20386
Seattle
Washington 98102, USA.
Tel 206 323 7610
Fax 206 323 7612

American Holistic Medical Association
6728 Old McLean Village Drive
McLean, VA 22101, USA
Tel 703 556 9222

American Academy of Medical Preventics
6151 West Century Boulevard, Suite 1114
Los Angeles
California 90045, USA.
Tel 213 645 5350

Eczema Association for Science and Education
1221 South West Yamhill, Suite 303
Portland
Oregon 97205, USA.
Tel 503 228 4430

Canadian Holistic Medical Association
700 Bay Street
PO Box 101, Suite 604
Toronto
Ontario M5G 1Z6, Canada.
Tel 416 599 0447

SOUTH AFRICA

South African Homoeopaths, Chiropractors & Allied Professions Board
PO Box 17055
0027 Gooenkloof
South Africa.
Tel 2712 466 455

UK & EUROPE

National Eczema Society
Tavistock House East
Tavistock Square
London WC1H 9RA.
Tel 071-388 4097
Registered charity. Membership costs £12 a year and subscribers

receive an information pack on managing eczema, a quarterly magazine giving details of the latest advances in treatment, support from local groups and meetings, and free access to the NES's Information Service.

British Complementary Medicine Association
St Charles Hospital
Exmoor Street
London W10 6DZ.
Tel 081-964 1205
Fax 081-964 1207
Umbrella organization representing organizations outside CCAM (below).

Council for Complementary and Alternative Medicine
179 Gloucester Place
London NW1 6DX.
Tel 071-724 9103
Fax 071-724 5330
Umbrella body representing professional organizations for acupuncture, herbal medicine, homoeopathy, osteopathy, chiropractic and naturopathy. Offer general information and direction to relevant organizations. For information leaflets on the main therapies send an sae and a cheque for £1.

Centre for Complementary Health Studies
University of Exeter
Streatham Court
Rennes Drive
Exeter, Devon EX4 4PU.
Tel 0392 264498

University-based research and
training in natural therapies. Offers
postgraduate studies, public lectures
and referral to approved practitioner
organizations.

Centre for the Study of
Complementary Medicine
51 Bedford Place
Southampton
Hampshire SO1 2DG
Tel 0703 334752
Also at
14 Harley House
Upper Harley Street
Off Marylebone Road
London NW1 4PR
Tel 071-935 7848
*Private centre staffed by medically
qualified and natural therapists
offering a variety of therapies
including acupuncture,
homoeopathy, clinical ecology,
biofeedback, psychotherapy and
hypnosis. Concessions for people on
low incomes. Pioneered the approach
of clinical ecology to food and
chemical sensitivities in the UK.
Also encourages post-graduate
teaching and research in natural
therapy techniques for doctors.*

Disability Alliance
Universal House
Wentworth Street
London E1 7SA.
Tel 071-247 8776
*Voluntary organization offering help
and advice on industrial
compensation. Write in or call the
Benefit and Rights Enquiries line
071-247 8763 (2 - 4pm Mon/Tues,
10.30 - 12.30 Thurs).*

Institute for Complementary
Medicine
PO Box 194
London SE16 1QZ
Tel 071-237 5165
Fax 071-237 5175
*Umbrella organization for those
outside BCMA and CCAM (above).*

Council for Acupuncture
179 Gloucester Place
London NW1 6DX.
071-724 5756
*Umbrella organization representing
major acupuncture bodies in the
UK. Offers general advice about
acupuncture and a directory of UK
practitioners for £2.*

British Medical Acupuncture
Association
Newton House
Newton Lane
Lower Whitley
Warrington
Cheshire WA4 4JA
Tel 0925-730727
*Membership limited to doctors,
dentists and vets trained in
acupuncture. Contact for names of
local practitioners.*

British Homoeopathic
Association
27a Devonshire Street
London W1N 1RJ.
Send sae for list of practitioners.

British Association for Counselling
1 Regent Place
Rugby
Warwickshire CV21 2PJ
Tel 0788-578328
Supply area lists of counsellors and organizations, fact-sheets and information on training. Send an sae.

British Society of Medical and Dental Hypnosis
42 Links Road
Ashtead
Surrey KT21 2HJ.
Tel 0372 273522.
All members are doctors or dentists trained in hypnotherapy. Call for details of local practitioners in London and south east or referral to regional offices throughout the country.

Register of Chinese Herbal Medicine
PO Box 400
Wembley
Middlesex HA9 9NZ
Tel 081-904 1357
Supplies lists of practitioners nationwide for £1.50 (cheque/PO) and A5 sae.

The Chi Centre
Riverbank House
Putney Bridge Approach
Fulham
London SW6 3JD
Tel 071-371 9717
Specializes in traditional Chinese herbal medicine for skin conditions, including the break-through 'cure' mentioned in this book. Staffed by doctors trained in both traditional Chinese and conventional medicine. Uses Western medicine as well, with counselling and free information. Free helpline number as above.

Useful further reading

The Greening of Medicine, Dr Patrick Pietroni (Gollancz, UK, 1990)

Medicine and Culture, Lynn Payer (Gollancz, UK, 1990)

The Alternative Dictionary of Symptoms and Cures, Dr Caroline Shreeve (Century, UK, 1987)

The Encyclopaedia of Alternative Health Care, Kristen Olsen (Piatkus, UK, 1989)

Acupuncture for Everyone, Dr Ruth Lever (Penguin, UK, 1987)

60-Second Shiatsu, Eva Shaw (Simon & Schuster, USA, 1990)

The Book of Shiatsu, Paul Lundberg (Gaia, UK, 1992)

Aromatherapy: Massage with Essential Oils, Christine Wildwood (Element, UK, 1991)

Flower Remedies, Christine Wildwood (Element, UK, 1991)

Clinical Ecology, Dr George Lewith and Dr Julian Kenyon (Thorsons, UK, 1985)

The Illustrated Herbal Handbook for Everyone, Juliette de Bairacli Levy (Faber & Faber, UK, 1991)

Herbs for Common Ailments, Anne McIntyre (Gaia, UK, 1992)

Evening Primrose, Kathryn Marsden (Vermillion, UK, 1993)

The Family Health Guide to Homoeopathy, Dr Barry Rose (Dragon's World, UK, 1992)

Homoeopathy: The Family Handbook, British Homoeopathic Association (Thorsons, UK, 1992)

A-Z of Natural Healthcare, Belinda Grant (Optima, UK, 1993)

An Encyclopaedia of Natural Medicine, Michael Murray and Joseph Pizzorno (Optima, UK, 1990)

Nutritional Medicine, Dr Stephen Davies and Dr Alan Stewart (Pan, UK, 1987)

The Stress Protection Plan, Leon Chaitow (Thorsons, UK, 1992)

Stressmanship, Dr Audrey Livingstone Booth (Severn House, UK, 1985)

Massage: A Practical Introduction, Stewart Mitchell (Element, UK, 1992)

Mind, Stress and Health, Dr Richard Totman (Condor, UK, 1990)

Against Therapy, Jeffrey Masson (Collins, UK, 1989)

Reflexology: Foot Massage for Total Health, Inge Dougans with Suzanne Ellis (Element, UK, 1991)

Reflexology, Chris Stormer (Headway/Hodder & Stoughton, UK, 1992)

The Illustrated Light on Yoga, B K S Iyengar (Aquarian/Thorsons, UK, 1993)

Index